The
Endometriosis
SURVIVAL
GUIDE

**Your guide to
the latest
treatment options
and the best
coping strategies**

Margot Joan Fromer

New Harbinger Publications

Publisher's Note

Distributed in the U.S.A. by Publishers Group West; in Canada by Raincoast Books; in Great Britain by Airlift Book Company, Ltd.; in South Africa by Real Books, Ltd.; in Australia by Boobook; and in New Zealand by Tandem Press.

Copyright © 1998 by Margot Joan Fromer
New Harbinger Publications, Inc.
5674 Shattuck Avenue
Oakland, CA 94609

Cover design © 1998 by Lightbourne Images.
Edited by Mary Lee Cole.
Text design by Michele Waters.

Library of Congress Catalog Card Number: 98-66707
ISBN 1-57224-152-7 Paperback

New Harbinger Publications' Website address: www.newharbinger.com

First printing

Contents

Introduction

Endometriosis is probably one of the most widely misunderstood of all the ailments that befall women. In fact, not much more is known about it today than in 1921 when endometriosis was first recognized and named. Not only do women themselves have an unclear idea of what endometriosis is, their doctors have trouble recognizing and treating it.

No one knows exactly how or why endometriosis occurs, or whether it is a separate disease or the result of another unidentified problem. In this book we will view it as a separate disease because most knowledgeable gynecologists treat it as a disease—and because, for all the physical, social, and emotional trouble it causes, it surely feels like one.

What Is Endometriosis?

Simply stated, although it is by no means a simple disease, endometriosis is the growth of normal endometrial tissue in an abnormal place. Endometriosis occurs when part of the lining of the uterus, called the endometrium, ends up in the abdominal cavity, perched on other organs or structures such as the outside of the uterus, the bladder, the large intestine, or the ovaries. And since the tissue itself is normal, it acts the same way that the correctly placed endometrium does: It builds up and then bleeds every month. This abnormally placed endometrial tissue, called endometrioma, has no way to release the blood it expels, so the blood stays within the abdominal cavity and causes pain, cramps, and other problems and symptoms (see chapter 2).

Just as women vary tremendously in the amount of discomfort they experience during a normal menstrual cycle, women with endometriosis experience a wide range in intensity of symptoms, from highly controllable with mild analgesics to devastating and life altering.

Diagnosis of endometriosis can be difficult, as many physicians have had little experience with it. Some of the more insecure ones even blame women for their own incompetence by telling them that the symptoms are all in their head. Moreover, medical treatment varies so widely, and there has been so little research on endometriosis and its causes, that it may be difficult to find doctors who know how to advise you, especially in rural areas and small towns. And to make matters worse, your relationship with your gynecologist is one of the key factors in the successful treatment and management of endometriosis.

Who Gets the Disease?

It is estimated that about 15 percent of all American women have endometriosis (approximately 5 million women), but the actual number is probably far higher because so many cases remain undiagnosed for two major reasons. First, many physicians do not recognize endometriosis and often confuse it with pelvic inflammatory disease, pelvic chlamydia infection, tubal pregnancy, premenstrual syndrome, endosalpingosis (inflammation of the fallopian tubes), and other abnormalities of the female reproductive tract. Second, some women either don't think to report pain and abnormal symptoms to their physicians or are afraid to. Some feel squeamish about talking about "female troubles," and others think that pain associated with their menstrual cycles is just an unavoidable part of being a woman.

Your Relationship with Your Physician

There are several effective treatments for endometriosis, including hormonal drugs and surgery, but the social and psychological effects of the disease are another story. Your relationship with your physician is key in overcoming endometriosis. Often it can be an uphill battle just getting your doctor to take seriously your complaints of severe pain that is not really menstrual pain, but pain that occurs in conjunction with menstruation (and at other times during the menstrual cycle). Stories abound of women whose doctors didn't pay attention to them, just plain didn't believe them, wouldn't listen to them, or didn't think the pain meant anything.

Some physicians who do recognize the problem as endometriosis recommend getting pregnant: "Just let your husband get you pregnant, dear, and all your troubles will be over." This "solution" can be one of the most cavalier and humiliating things that can happen to a woman with endometriosis. Not only is it a terrible reason for making the all-important decision to have a child, it is an irresponsible suggestion. Although endometriosis does indeed go into remission during pregnancy, the disease comes right back after delivery—sometimes worse than ever.

Being treated like this may be something women have grown accustomed to over years of dealing with physicians, but that doesn't make it any easier to bear. It makes you angry. It makes you question the reality of the pain—even though you *know* it hurts like hell. When a doctor looks at you, literally or figuratively pats you on the head, and says, "It's nothing. Just live with it," you may feel hurt and powerless. Many women at that point run to another doctor who may say the same thing. See chapter 5 and chapter 9 for ways to cope with this stress and to improve your relationship with your physician.

Such a wide range of symptoms and such differing degrees of pain make it hard to talk to your friends about what you're experiencing. It's also hard to get a sufficient handle on your symptoms to discuss them with your doctor because some months the pain is just terrible and some months it's not too bad. And what's worse, there's usually no way to predict when it will increase in severity, although endometriosis usually gets progressively worse over the years if it remains untreated.

The physical and emotional pain of endometriosis is compounded by the fact that it doesn't "show." You look healthy, therefore it is difficult for people to believe that you have a chronic, sometimes debilitating condition, often dubbed "the great gynecological crippler." Moreover, endometriosis is never life threatening, so it's easy for other people to dismiss it as less than serious. "Just be glad you don't have something *really* bad like cancer."

Endometriosis is an expensive disease. You will have to purchase medication, perhaps have surgery, and sooner or later you are bound to lose time from work, maybe even to the extent of jeopardizing your job. Unfortunately, endometriosis disrupts your life in a number of ways, and if the pain is severe, you might not be able to function well for a few days each month. This gets very tedious very quickly. You may bleed more during your menstrual period and have bleeding between periods. This gets old, too. Your sex life will be negatively affected to some extent, and men vary in their willingness to be understanding about this.

Myths and Misperceptions

You've probably bought this book because you have endometriosis or someone close to you has it. Chances are this isn't the first time you've heard the word endometriosis, but like most people, you're not sure exactly what it means and what having the disease entails.

Chances are too that many of the things about endometriosis that you do know, or that you *think* you know, are wrong. For example:

- Endometriosis is *not* a disease of thin, white women who have never been married, or at least have never had children. The truth is that, although it is more common in women in their thirties and forties, any woman can get the disease, regardless of race, religion, or ethnic group.

- Tampons do *not* cause endometriosis. The type of feminine protection you use to absorb menstrual flow has no bearing on your risk of the disease.

- Sexual intercourse during your period does *not* cause endometriosis. Feel free to have sex whenever you feel like it.

- Hysterectomy is *not* the only sure cure for endometriosis. There are many ways to treat the disease, and hysterectomy is one of the last on the list of things to try.

- Stress does *not* cause endometriosis. Although having the disease is stressful, as is having any disease, you didn't get it from worrying.

How to Use This Book

Depending on what you already know about endometriosis, and what you would like to learn, you can read this book straight through from beginning to end, or you can pick and choose among the chapters.

If you have recently been diagnosed with endometriosis, you probably should start at the beginning because whatever your doctor has said will most likely be confusing, or you may have forgotten a good part of it. Moreover, whatever you heard in the doctor's office is not the entire story. This is not to say that doctors deliberately avoid giving their patients information (although it is true of some of them); rather, they cannot possibly cover the entire story of endometriosis at one visit—or even several.

Since you probably have about a million questions, read this book at your leisure, take notes if that helps you learn, and underline passages that you find particularly relevant. In other words, use the book as a both a learning tool and as a reference. The women whose stories and experiences with endometriosis are interspersed throughout this book are real people, but their names have been changed to protect their confidentiality. Some of their experiences will be similar to yours and some will not, but there is something to be learned from all of them because they have come to grips with, and even solved, a wide variety of problems that accompany endometriosis. In addition, these women's stories add a personal dimension to discussions of the diagnosis, treatment, and progress of the disease.

If you have had endometriosis for years, there will be some new ideas here for you, especially in the chapters on treatment and management of pain and stress (chapters 4, 5, and 6). You also might find things to think about regarding your relationships with physicians and the health care system.

Regardless of how you choose to read *The Endometriosis Survival Guide*, it was written with you in mind. Just as you are the only one who knows how badly and in what ways you are affected by the disease, you are the only one who can make the decision about how to use this book. However you choose to read it, use it to your best advantage—and be healthy.

Endometriosis at a Glance: Frequently Asked Questions

What is endometriosis?

Endometriosis is a disease characterized by misplaced endometrial tissue: migration of the endometrium from where it belongs in the uterus to where it does not—on the ovaries, fallopian tubes, and other pelvic and abdominal organs and structures.

Is the incidence of endometriosis increasing?

Possibly. It is diagnosed more often, so the numbers are greater. Also, women know more about endometriosis now and discuss it more openly; therefore, because women talk about it more, it seems as if there are more cases. There is no way to know, however, how many women actually have the disease—probably more than five million in the United States. Some people put the figure at 25–30 percent of all women.

What are the symptoms?

Pain is the most common symptom. Others include changes in menstrual pattern, changes in bowel function, backache, and infertility.

What causes the disease?

No one knows for sure. The most likely theory is retrograde menstruation; that is, some menstrual fluid backs up into the pelvic cavity instead of it all being released to the outside during the monthly flow. There are other theories as well: spread of endometrial cells via the lymphatic system or via the circulatory system; "escape" and spread of such cells as a result of surgery; and transformation of fetal tissue.

How is it diagnosed?

Definitive diagnosis is made only by laparoscopy. However, a pattern of symptoms and typical medical history will lead an astute physician to a strong suspicion of endometriosis.

What's a laparoscopy?

Laparoscopy consists of inserting a long, thin hollow tube into the abdominal cavity through a very small incision inside or very close to the navel. A light attached to fiberoptic bundles is then threaded through the tube so the surgeon can see the inside of the abdomen.

How old are women who have endometriosis?

They are usually in their childbearing years. The age range when endometriosis is most common is twenty to forty, although it is possible to get the disease as early as menarche and as late as menopause.

How is the disease classified?

The American Fertility Society has divided endometriosis into four stages, from minimal to severe, depending on the number, location, and depth of endometriomata.

Did I get endometriosis from using tampons?

No, there is no evidence to suggest that.

Did I get endometriosis from having sex during my period?

No.

Is it catching?

No.

Do menstrual cramps cause endometriosis?

No. Pain during menstruation is a result, not a cause, of endometriosis.

Is it inherited?

Possibly. There is certainly a familial tendency to endometriosis, but just because your mother had it does not mean that you automatically will. However, when the disease is familial, it tends to be more severe.

Does putting off childbirth until after age thirty cause endometriosis?

It doesn't cause the disease but it may contribute to the severity. The more menstrual periods a woman has, the more likely it is that the disease will increase in severity.

I've heard that if I get pregnant my endometriosis will go away. Is this true?

It *may*, but there's no guarantee. And the disease will probably come right back after you have your baby. Also, sometimes endometriosis gets worse during pregnancy, and anyway, having endometriosis is not a good reason to have a baby. There are better and more effective treatments.

Will my endometriosis go away after menopause?

Probably, but there's no guarantee.

Do teenage girls get endometriosis?

Yes, but it's rare.

Why are the ovaries the common site for endometriosis?

Because they are on the direct route of retrograde menstruation, and endometrial tissue tends to land there first and implant. Fallopian tubes are another common site for the same reason.

Are some women more prone to the disease than others?

Yes, women who have never been pregnant. The disease is less common in women with an irregular menstrual cycle or who do not ovulate every month. Women who have interrupted their cycles by taking birth control pills or by frequent pregnancies seem less at risk for the disease.

Why do women with endometriosis get adhesions? What are they?

Adhesions are bands of scar tissue that cause surfaces of organs and tissues to adhere to one another instead of remaining separated as they normally should. Adhesions are common after abdominal surgery. In women with endometriosis, adhesions also are common perhaps because the backflow of menstrual blood and endometrial tissue produces irritation and inflammation in the pelvic cavity, which eventually causes a buildup of scar tissue.

What's the cure for endometriosis?

Endometriosis can't be "cured" in the sense that an infection is cured by a dose of antibiotics. It is treated either by surgery to remove the endometriomata or by a variety of hormonal drugs and analgesics.

My friend said her endometriosis went away when she started taking birth control pills. Should I believe her?

Yes. The same combination of estrogen and progesterone found in oral contraceptive pills is one of the several treatments for endometriosis.

I've heard that danazol is a "miracle drug" for endometriosis. Is that true?

Danazol, a synthetic androgen (male hormone), can be very effective in treating endometriosis, but there are no miracle cures for the disease.

Isn't taking hormones bad for you?

Not if you take them in the proper dosage for a certain amount of time. All drugs have side effects, but those you may get from the hormonal drugs used to treat endometriosis are usually mild and not dangerous. If the side effects bother you, however, you can stop taking them.

Are some women at higher risk for endometriosis than others?

There's debate about this. It may be that women who are obese, smoke cigarettes, and abuse drugs and alcohol are at higher risk for endometriosis-related infertility, but no one knows this for certain.

Is it possible to prevent the disease?

Maybe. There's debate about this too, and there's no proof one way or another, because no one knows what causes endometriosis in the first place.

1

Female Reproductive Anatomy and Physiology

You may be tempted to skip over this chapter if you think it will be dry and technical. But not only is the information it contains easy to understand, you should know something about the workings of your reproductive organs and structures. It's good to learn a little about your own anatomy and physiology and even more important, the knowledge will come in handy when you talk with your physician about endometriosis. The more you know about the disease, the better able you will be to understand and manage it.

Anatomy

External Organs and Structures

Female pelvic structures have two major purposes: reproduction and sexual pleasure. The *vulva* (also known as the pudendum) comprises the external genitalia, consisting of:

- The *labia majora* are two folds of fatty tissue, from which pubic hair arises, that enclose and protect the structures that lie behind them.

- The *labia minora* are two thinner folds of tissue, not covered by hair, behind the labia majora. They are richly endowed with nerve endings and blood vessels and thus highly responsive to sexual stimulation. They extend from the clitoral hood to the top of the perineum.

- Just behind the labia minora is the *vestibule*, which contains two separate orifices—one to the urethra (the tube leading from the bladder through which urine passes to the outside), and the other to the vagina.

- *Bartholin's glands* lie at either side of the opening to the vagina and are responsible for lubrication during sexual excitement.

- The *clitoris* is located at the top of the inverted V formed by the labia minora. Its sole purpose is initiating and elevating levels of sexual excitement. It is the only structure in the human body that has pleasure as its sole purpose. (Men have no analogous structure.)

The *vagina* is the canal leading from the vulva to the cervix (see Internal Organs and Structures and figure 1–b on the next page). It has three main functions: sexual intercourse, the passageway for the outflow of menstrual fluid, and the birth canal. Unless it is being used for intercourse or birth, the canal is collapsed on itself. It stretches to accommodate a penis or a fetus.

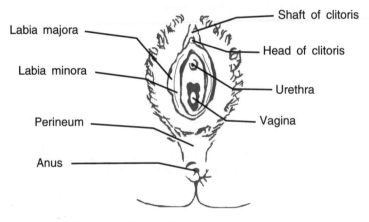

Figure 1–a. External Pelvic Organs

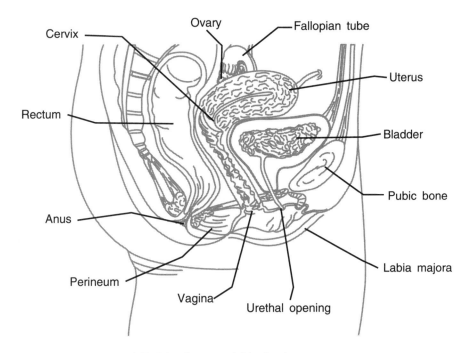

Figure 1–b. Internal Pelvic Organs (sideview)

Internal Organs and Structures

The rest of the female reproductive structures are internal (see figures 1–b and 1–c). The *uterus* is a hollow, pear-shaped organ a few inches long, designed to house and nourish a fetus during pregnancy. The uterus is made of tough muscle fibers that have an amazing ability to stretch and expand during pregnancy.

The neck of the uterus, which protrudes and opens into the vagina, is called the *cervix*. During labor, the cervix dilates from almost completely closed to wide enough to permit passage of a full-term infant.

The *endometrium* is the lining of the uterus and is composed of vascular tissue that is influenced by and responds to hormones. Each month, the endometrium thickens and becomes more vascular (rich in blood vessels) in preparation for a fertilized ovum (egg). If pregnancy does not occur, the endometrium is shed in the process known as menstruation. It is this tissue that is the source of all the trouble for women with endometriosis.

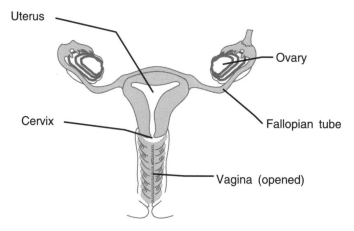

Figure 1–c.   Internal Pelvic Organs (frontview)

The *fallopian tubes* lead from the ovaries to the uterus, through which an ovum, or egg, passes and where it is met by sperm to be fertilized. The fertilized or unfertilized ovum then continues its journey down the tube to the uterus. The tubes are physically connected only to the uterus. At the other end (the fimbriated end), they lie close to the ovaries but are not actually attached. When an ovum is released from an ovary each month, it must jump across space (granted, a very tiny space) from the ovary into the fallopian tube.

The two *ovaries* are small organs about the size and shape of almonds that float (attached to the peritoneum only by ligaments) above the uterus. They secrete female sex hormones and produce ova.

Reproductive organs and structures are held in place by a variety of skeletal supports and ligaments (bands of strong fibrous connective tissue). The *bony pelvis* is composed of two innominate bones, the *sacrum* and the *coccyx*. Each innominate bone contains three parts: *ilium, ischium,* and *pubis*. These bones form an arch around and protect the internal reproductive organs and are designed to protect the developing fetus.

Four pairs of *ligaments* support the uterus, ovaries, and fallopian tubes, and a variety of blood vessels and nerves provide nourishment and neurologic function.

Physiology

Anatomy is the study of body structure, and physiology is the way those structures function and interact with one another. The physiology of the female reproductive system (the male system too, for that matter) is based on production and cyclical ebbing and flowing of hormones. The following account is a simplified synopsis of a highly complex system, which you really don't have to master in order to understand endometriosis. It is included here as an extra for women who want to know more about how their bodies function. It is here also in case you have questions about some of the terms and descriptions your doctor uses and you want to look them up when you get home, or in case you want to refer to them as you learn more about endometriosis.

The Menstrual Cycle

The *menstrual cycle*, with which we are all familiar, is divided into three hormone dependent phases: *follicular*, *ovulation*, and *luteal* (see figure 1–d). Hormones are chemical substances produced by endocrine glands that regulate various body processes. The following glands and other structures are of special importance to the female reproductive system:

- The *hypothalamus* is the part of the brain that connects the nervous and endocrine systems. It transmits messages between the two and controls secretion of hormones from the pituitary gland. The hypothalamus also controls body temperature.

- The *pituitary gland*, the master gland that governs the entire menstrual cycle, is located at the base of the brain and is connected to the hypothalamus. It coordinates the secretion of various hormones.

- Hormones secreted by the ovaries are *estrogen*, which, among its many functions, stimulates the growth of the endometrium, and *progesterone*, which matures and prepares the endometrium for the fertilized ovum.

- *Gonadotropins* are pituitary hormones that stimulate the ovaries.

- *Gonadotropin-releasing hormones* are neurochemical trans-
  mitters sent by the hypothalamus to direct release of gonadotropins.

During the *follicular phase*, hormones, particularly *follicle
stimulating hormone (FSH)*, a gonadotropin released by the pituitary gland, trigger the growth of the follicle within an ovary. A
follicle is the basic functional unit of the ovary, the source of both
ova and hormones. Each month a follicle begins to grow, and this
initial follicular growth ends with a detectable rise in estrogen. As
the follicle continues to mature it produces increasing levels of estrogen, reaching a peak at ovulation. FSH declines as estrogen
rises, but *luteinizing hormone (LH)*, another gonadotropin, increases
steadily.

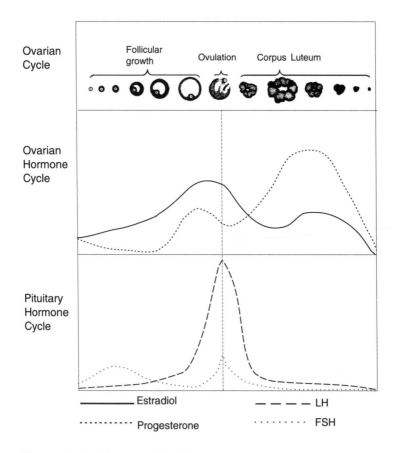

Figure 1–d. Hormonal Cycles

Ovulation occurs when a mature ovum is released from the ovary. A rise in estradiol (a type of estrogen) sets off a gonadotropin surge in midcycle, and the gonadotropin-releasing hormone (GnRH) causes an increase in both LH and FSH. LH brings about ovulation, and FSH assists in production of the corpus luteum, a structure formed by the ruptured follicle. The follicle ruptures within twenty-four hours after the LH peak, and it is believed that physical expulsion of the ovum results from an increase in a prostaglandin (a nonhormonal chemical produced by various body tissues) triggered by LH.

Immediately after ovulation, the fimbriated end of a fallopian tube takes hold of the released ovum and draws it into the tube, where it is propelled by wave-like contractions (much like those that pass matter along the digestive tract) into the uterus. The trip takes about four or five days, and along the way, the ovum may be fertilized if there are viable sperm in the tube.

After the follicle ruptures, certain cells increase in size and accumulate lutein to form the *corpus luteum* out of the ruptured follicle. Eight or nine days after ovulation, the corpus luteum is filled with blood vessels and is associated with peak levels of progesterone and estradiol. It also produces other hormones called androgens, as well as estrogens and progestins. Ten to twelve days after ovulation, if fertilization of the ovum has not occurred, the corpus luteum begins to regress. If fertilization has occurred, the corpus luteum produces human chorionic gonadotropin (HCG), which maintains the corpus luteum until the pregnancy is firmly established at about nine or ten weeks.

If there is no pregnancy and the corpus luteum keeps regressing, estrogen and progesterone levels diminish to a point where the endometrium cannot be maintained and it sloughs off as menstruation.

Uterine Cycle

The *uterine cycle* consists of two phases: *proliferative* phase and *secretory* phase. In the proliferative phase, estrogen influences the endometrium to grow and increase in thickness. Cervical glands also step up secretions and the vaginal lining thickens somewhat. As a result of the developing corpus luteum, progesterone causes secretory changes in the endometrium that result in changes in its appearance and function; that is, it becomes thicker and more vascular. The major purpose of this phase is to provide a "bed" for the fertilized ovum.

For many centuries and in many cultures, *menstruation*, the secretory phase, has been described by women as the "weeping of a disappointed uterus"—or some similar expression. If the ovum is not fertilized and thus does not implant on the endometrium, hormones influence prostaglandins to constrict the tightly coiled small arteries that have developed as the endometrium thickened. The constricted arteries bleed, taking along sluffed-off endometrium. Menstrual flow lasts two to eight days and consists of blood, endometrial tissue, and cervical and vaginal mucus.

There have always been lots of taboos and myths surrounding menstruation, and women themselves have contributed to its "bad press." We have called it all sorts of negative and unflattering names: the "curse," being "on the rag," the "red tide," and far worse.

In pagan times (and even today in some societies that we consider less enlightened than our own), menstruating women have been shunned, cast out of their homes, and even buried in the ground up to their necks the entire time they were menstruating. Most religions have treated menstruating women as less than desirable, and some have considered them unclean and downright harmful. For example, the most orthodox and traditional branches of some Western religions do not allow women at the altar lest they be menstruating.

Things are only slightly better today. Although it is not politically correct among educated, socially advanced people to discriminate against women because they menstruate, the following are some of the negative beliefs and stereotypes that won't go away:

- A menstruating woman should stay away from other people as much as possible.

- She should curtail her physical activity while she has her period, and she certainly should not engage in sexual activity.

- Women are particularly moody and emotionally unstable while they are menstruating, and they have difficulty functioning normally at work.

- A woman has trouble thinking clearly while she is menstruating.
- Menstrual pain is all in the mind, that is, it isn't real.

It's not just men who handicap us by believing—and acting on—these myths and stereotypes. Many times, women are their own worst enemies when it comes to taboos about menstruation. Most of us have been taught that it's not nice or ladylike to talk about our menstrual periods, or sexual function, or any of that other "nasty stuff." So no wonder we have trouble acknowledging that something is wrong. Going to a doctor who will make us talk about it in detail, and then submit us to an examination, is excruciatingly embarrassing to most of us.

2

Definition and Causes of Endometriosis

Endometriosis is a condition in which some endometrial tissue grows in parts of the body other than inside the uterus where it belongs. It usually settles somewhere in the lower abdominal cavity, most commonly on the outside of the uterus, or on the ovaries, fallopian tubes, or uterine ligaments. Endometrial tissue may also be found on the large intestine, urinary bladder and even, in very rare instances, in the arms, legs, or head.

Endometrial tissue that has migrated from the inside of the uterus to other areas of the body where it does not occur naturally is called *endometrioma* (the plural is endometriomata), *endometrial nodules, endometrial lesions,* and *endometrial growths*— these four terms all mean the same thing.

Relatively little medical research has been done on endometriosis though ironically it is one of the most common gynecological diseases.

Endometriosis does not occur prior to *menarche* (a woman's first menstrual period), it is rare in women under age twenty and after menopause, although it has been known to recur in menopausal women who take hormone replacement therapy. The disease is most common in women age twenty-three to forty, and there are no racial differences in the incidence and prevalence of endometriosis. A tendency toward the disease may be inherited, and if a close blood relative (mother or sister) has the disease, you are more likely to have it, too. No gene or gene marker has yet been found for endometriosis, but it is likely that one exists because the frequency of the disease within families is higher than exists in the general population.

Linda, one of the women I interviewed, is one of those unlucky women who has had endometriosis from the time she first began to menstruate, although for ages, she didn't know what it was. She was thirteen or fourteen when she got her first period, and the cramps started right away. "None of my friends were in as much pain as I was," she said. "I couldn't believe how much it hurt."

She's twenty-one now and her face screws up in horror as she remembers the way it was when she was a teenager. Were the cramps bad enough to have to miss school? "Oh, my God," she recalls, "missing school was the least of it. Lying in bed all curled up with a heating pad and bottles of Motrin. It was awful."

Linda thinks her mother probably has endometriosis, too, based on the way she behaves when she has her period; however, they never discuss it.

"That's one of the big problems," says Linda. "I can't talk to my mom about it. I don't really talk to her about anything, but there's no other woman I'm close to, so I've had to go through the whole thing pretty much alone—the surgery and everything."

Linda's father has taken her to the emergency room a few times when the pain has been unendurable, "But your dad isn't really the one you want at a time like that. He's been great—real gentle and nice, but still ..."

A father is a man, and a young girl, now a young woman, needs another woman to lean on when she's in the throes of "female troubles."

There is some speculation that the incidence of endometriosis might be increasing, at least in North America and Western Europe. This could be perception rather than reality since awareness of the disease is on the rise, and physicians are becoming somewhat more sophisticated about diagnosing it. Then again, the reported increased incidence may be real because of changing menstrual patterns. Many women are postponing childbirth until their thirties and forties, thus they have significantly more menstrual periods than women did several decades ago, presenting many more opportunities for endometrial tissue to migrate outside the uterus.

Signs and Symptoms

Endometriosis causes a wide range of symptoms and other phenomena. Because the disease consists of normal endometrial tissue that is abnormally placed, it behaves as it "should" by building up in response to hormonal influences and by bleeding at the time of the menstrual period, but because the bloody shedding of this tissue is in an *abnormal* place, it has no way to leave the body. The result is internal bleeding, inflammation, and formation of cysts and scar tissue. This process, which occurs every month, causes pain, the severity of which depends on the location of the endometriomata. It may or may not have anything to do with the size of the lesions.

Therefore, pain at the time of menstruation is the most common symptom of endometriosis and is usually what brings a woman to an obstetrician gynecologist (OBG) for help.

Many of the women with endometriosis that I interviewed said they experienced severe menstrual pain from the very beginning. Avis said she was "doubled over every month right from day one." So did Lorraine—she used the term "doubled over in pain" as well. Both women described missing days of school because of excruciating menstrual cramps, often accompanied by nausea and vomiting. One day, things were so bad that Lorraine's father had to come to school to take her home. "He didn't like having to leave work, and I was so embarrassed I thought I'd die," she said.

But Jean was fine until her late twenties. Her menarche was at age twelve, and for about fifteen years, things were normal. Then she began experiencing the symptoms that so many of the other women described: pain every month that was an eight or nine on a scale of ten. Jean said that she thought her endometriosis was complicated by a uterine fibroid tumor (myoma), a normally painless and benign growth in the uterine musculature.

Endometriosis has been dubbed "benign cancer" because of the way it spreads to distant sites (akin to the metastasis of cancer), and then attaches to and invades organs and structures to which it does not belong. However, it is *not* a malignant disease and does *not* consume and destroy those organs and structures. In *very* rare instances (less than 1 percent of all women with endometriosis), the disease does turn malignant, as a low-grade cancer known as *adenoacanthoma*, which usually does not spread and is rarely fatal.

Other symptoms include:

- pain at ovulation and sexual intercourse

- excessive or irregular menstrual bleeding

- midcycle bleeding (menstrual irregularity may be due to some of the organic causes or anatomical dysfunction that causes the endometriosis in the first place)

- higher-than-average risk of natural abortion (miscarriage)

- infertility

- ruptured ovarian cysts (called "chocolate cysts" because of the old blood they contain)

- adhesions

- increased risk of ectopic pregnancy

- alterations in bowel movements (constipation or diarrhea, or both)

- various intestinal upsets

- urinary frequency

- pain on urination

- lower backache

In addition, rupture of large endometriomata can cause massive bleeding into the abdominal cavity, which is a surgical emergency.

Nature of the Symptoms

In general, the type of symptoms you have depends on the location of the endometrial lesions. For instance, if they have settled in your rectum or lower large bowel, you may be constipated and have pain when you move your bowels; you may experience urgency to defecate and have blood in your stool. If endometrial tissue has traveled to your fallopian tubes, you will likely be infertile, but if you do manage to get pregnant, you are at increased risk of ectopic pregnancy. And in the unlikely event that you have endometriomata in your chest, you may have pain there or in your shoulder, and you may cough up blood.

If this seems like an incredibly broad, depressing, and scary range of symptoms, it is. The good news, however, is that the vast majority of women with endometriosis do not suffer from them all, and many experience no symptoms at all—or at least such mild ones that they don't suspect anything is amiss.

Pain is not only the most common symptom, it is the most worrisome and the one that women dread the most. Chapter 3 will provide details of what you can do to counteract, alleviate, and bear the pain, but suffice it to say here that the severity of the pain is not necessarily related to the severity of the disease, that is, the number and size of the endometriomata. It is a medical conundrum that tiny endometriomata called *petechial growths* can produce more prostaglandins than larger ones. Prostaglandins are naturally occurring chemicals derived from fatty acids that have a variety of functions and are believed to be implicated in the pain of endometriosis.

Now that you feel thoroughly depressed by this litany of symptoms, you should know that one of the reasons that endometriosis is so often misdiagnosed is that the symptoms it manifests are similar to those of a wide range of other gynecologic conditions and diseases: adenomyosis (invasion of the uterine musculature by endometrial tissue), appendicitis, benign ovarian cysts, bowel obstruction, colon and ovarian cancers, diverticulitis, ectopic pregnancy, fibroid tumors of the uterus, gonorrhea, inflammatory bowel disease, irritable bowel syndrome, pelvic inflammatory disease, and others.

Helen had symptoms of endometriosis from the time she began to menstruate at eleven years of age until she had a hysterectomy at age forty. She's forty-six now. That's a long time to suffer without knowing why.

"By the time I had my third menstrual period, I had agonizing cramps every month. When I was in my twenties and thirties, I sometimes had to spend a day in bed when I had my period. The bad pain lasted two or three days every month, and I often lost that many days of work because I could hardly stand up straight.

At the time, I had a woman boss, and she was much nastier about my menstrual cramps than a man would have been. Apparently she never had a moment's trouble with her periods and thought that I was just 'a complaining female.' But one day I fainted at my desk and then she had to take me seriously."

Helen described this experience quietly and with very little emotion. Did she ever mention the pain to a gynecologist? "Oh God, yes! Every time I went to a new OBG—and I've had about five or six of them, men and women—they all said, 'Just live with it.' At one point, someone prescribed Motrin and Naprosyn [two kinds of nonsteroidal anti-inflammatory drugs], but they made me sleepy."

But did they help the pain? Helen acknowledged that the drugs were helpful, but she said it reluctantly. "I always felt as though my doctors wouldn't take the endometriosis seriously if an ordinary drug relieved some of the pain."

Twenty years before she finally had a hysterectomy (for fibroid tumors, not for the endometriosis, which wasn't diagnosed until the operation), Helen took oral contraceptives for three years. The symptoms abated somewhat during that time, but she began to read "horror stories" about birth control pills, stopped taking them, and had an intrauterine device (IUD) inserted. That didn't last long because she then read about the dangers of IUDs and had hers removed.

After that, she used other barrier birth control methods. "But there were a few times when I had unprotected sex, and that's when I thought I might be infertile."

Social and Psychological Symptoms

In addition to physical symptoms, endometriosis has other consequences. The chronicity, and steadily increasing severity with age, can result in feelings of debilitation, depression, and hopelessness. Many women are unable to carry on their normal lives for two or three days each month, sometimes longer. They can't work or take care of their personal lives, and they don't want to have sex. This gets *very* old *very* quickly. In other words, endometriosis can be a highly disruptive disease that will continue, if left untreated, until menopause.

Although there is no absolute cure for endometriosis in the sense that the disease disappears to the point where you might never have had it, there are highly effective treatments, so if you think you have the disease, make an appointment immediately with your OBG and get it diagnosed and treated. There is no reason for you to continue to suffer.

Causes of Endometriosis

Retrograde Transportation

There are two major theories about the cause of endometriosis. The first is *retrograde transportation* of the endometrium. This is believed to occur by spontaneous implantation of endometrial tissue that moves backward from the uterus through the fallopian tubes into the peritoneum (abdominal cavity) via reflux menstrual flow.

Three or perhaps more phenomena may be at work here. First is poor immunologic resistance; that is, the immune system fails to treat the floating endometrial cells as foreign invaders, and they are then accepted as host tissue and allowed to implant. Some monkeys were found to have an immunologic tolerance to endometrial tissue, but no one seems to know whether the deficiency in immunologic cells existed before the development of endometriosis or as a result of implantation of endometrial tissue outside the uterus (Reprogen, Inc., 1997).

The second phenomenon is the action of prostaglandins, which is still poorly understood. Third, it is possible that endometrial tissue moves from the uterus to other parts of the body through the lymph or blood systems.

Whatever the underlying cause, retrograde transportation causes endometrial tissue to implant first on the outside of the uterus and then metastasize from there. Support for this theory is derived from a number of factors:

- Endometriosis is most common on the ovaries, which are in the direct path of menstruation.

- Endometriosis is strongly correlated with an abnormally positioned uterus. For example, if the uterus is tipped forward, endometriomata are commonly found in the anterior pelvis, and if it is tipped backward, the endometriomata are found in the posterior pelvis.

• Women who have other anatomic abnormalities, such as cervical stenosis (narrowing of the cervix), absence of a cervix, imperforate hymen, and transverse vaginal septum (a vagina that is divided lengthwise by a membrane, much like the nose is divided into two nostrils), are more likely to develop endometriosis.

Endometriosis often waxes and wanes throughout a woman's reproductive years, but if it is left untreated, the general trend seems to be worsening of the disease. This makes sense if the cause is indeed retrograde transportation because each menstrual period offers renewed opportunity for endometriomata to establish themselves. Moreover, constant and repeated hormonal stimulation encourages the misplaced tissue to proliferate and burrow deeper into pelvic organs and structures.

However, until more definitive research is done, there is no way to be certain how fast the disease progresses, or if steadily worsening symptoms are due to increased numbers and size of endometriomata or to an entirely different (but most likely related) phenomenon.

Transformation of Tissue

The other major causation theory is *transformation of endometrial tissue*. Transformation may be a result of the mutation capabilities of endometrial tissue. Any tissue that arises out of fetal colonic tissue (that which develops into the large intestine) can later differentiate into endometrium-like tissue. In other words, the propensity toward endometriosis originated when you were still a fetus and the tissue that eventually developed into your colon underwent mutation. After menarche (the onset of menstruation), it was somehow stimulated by factors such as inflammation, infection, or endocrine imbalance.

This theory is less popular than retrograde transportation, probably because it doesn't make as much physiologic sense. The professional literature on endometriosis acknowledges the possibility of transformation of embryonic colonic tissue as a causative factor, but its likelihood is remote.

Inadvertent Implantation During Surgery

Another possibility about the cause of endometriosis is inadvertent implantation of endometrial tissue during uterine surgery. That is, endometrial tissue "escapes" from where it belongs and settles where it does not. This sounds highly logical, but has yet to be proven or disproven.

Redwine's Theory

David Redwine, M.D., an Oregon gynecologist, believes that endometriosis is congenital; that is, women are born with it. He also believes that the disease is not progressive but merely changes in appearance over time.

According to Redwine, during a female embryo's gestation, endometrial tissue develops from certain ducts in the pelvic cavity that differentiate into the various reproductive organs. He believes that not all endometrial cells make it to the uterus; some remain in the pelvis. During puberty, when hormones begin to kick in, the symptoms of endometriosis start, although Redwine says that the disease itself has little to do with reproductive hormonal fluctuations. Redwine's theory is almost indistinguishable from the transformation of tissue theory. He has several web sites on the Internet that you can visit to find a more detailed explanation of his theory.

Redwine's treatment, used by a number of other gynecologists around the country, is to remove a good deal of the peritoneum, where he believes most of the endometriomata are located. According to Redwine, the immediate postoperative success rate with this type of surgery is excellent, but because the cutting is so extensive, the risk of adhesions is high. This in turn increases the risk of disease recurrence. No studies have confirmed the long-term effects of Redwine's treatment—or the causation theory itself.

Yet another theory is called *angiogenesis*, the process by which body tissue creates new blood vessels. Angiogenesis is a new and increasingly popular explanation of the way cancer metastasizes, but it also has some scientists thinking about the development and spread of endometriosis. The ability of endometrial tissue to "set up housekeeping" outside the uterus depends on its ability to establish and maintain an adequate blood supply, i.e., angiogenesis. In recent studies, a newly discovered angiogenic growth factor has appeared in higher-than-normal quantities in the peritoneal fluid (the fluid that normally exists inside the peritoneal cavity) of women with endometriosis (Smith, 1997). Retrograde menstruation as well as activated macrophages (scavenger cells) may be two sources of this angiogenic growth factor.

Diagnosis

Endometriosis is definitively diagnosed by visualizing endometrial lesions using laparoscopy, a procedure in which the abdomen is distended with carbon dioxide gas and a tube is inserted through a small incision near or in the umbilicus (belly button). Attached to the tube is a light, and by moving the laparoscope around the abdomen, the physician can look at the abdominal organs to see if there are endometrial implants.

Even before using this surgical procedure, a good OBG can make a fairly accurate diagnosis by other means, although treatment really should not begin until a definitive diagnosis is made. Taking a detailed gynecologic history and asking appropriate questions usually results in a strong suspicion of endometriosis, because the pattern and nature of the symptoms have commonalities.

This is how Jean's disease was diagnosed. "I described my symptoms, and he did a colposcopy [which is not generally diagnostic of endometriosis] and put me on danazol, which helped the pain but gave me horrible side effects." As soon as Jean stopped the hormone drug danazol (more about this drug in chapter 4), the endometriosis returned, and when she was about thirty, she had a laparoscopy.

During a manual pelvic examination, the physician can often feel the lesions. No laboratory tests will confirm their presence, but doctors who have seen enough cases of endometriosis have a fairly good idea of what is going on. In addition, if other conditions that have similar symptoms—pelvic inflammatory disease, ectopic pregnancy, cysts, cancer, appendicitis and diverticulitis, for example—are ruled out, endometriosis can be pretty closely diagnosed by a process of elimination. However, your doctor cannot say for certain that you have endometriosis until the lesions are actually seen through a laparoscope.

Avis had a laparoscopy when she was twenty-two years old and had had undiagnosed endometriosis for eleven years. The procedure was mainly diagnostic, but the doctor told Avis that he had "burned out" some of the endometriomata. "That was when he told me I'd never get pregnant," she said. The prognosis turned out to be true, but the harshness and inflexibility of the statement was hard to take at the time. He also told her that there was no treatment for endometriosis.

If for some reason, you do not want to have a laparoscopy (although it is considered minor surgery and is usually done on an outpatient basis, it *is* an operation and you *will* have a very small scar), or your doctor feels it is not appropriate right now, ultrasonography often can reveal the presence of endometriomata.

Classification

The severity of endometriosis is classified according to four stages, and treatment is usually recommended based on the stage. The staging system was developed by the American Fertility Society (AFS) and uses a scale for the size, location, and number of endometrial lesions (ACOG, 1993).

The disadvantage of using only this system for choosing a treatment method is that it depends solely on visualization of the anatomical effects of the disease. It does not take into account other aspects such as degree of pain, amount of lifestyle disruption, factors that might have contributed to the endometriosis in the first place, and fluctuations in the size of the endometriomata.

According to the AFS, the higher the stage, the worse the disease and the greater the chance of infertility.

- Stage I (minimal) involves only the peritoneum and right ovary. The lesions are superficial.

- Stage II (mild) involves the peritoneum and both ovaries. The lesions are superficial or deep.

- Stage III (moderate) involves the peritoneum, cul-de-sac, both fallopian tubes, and both ovaries.

- Stage IV (severe) involves considerable disease in many or all locations.

Early and Late Endometriosis

Adolescence

Having said that endometriosis occurs mostly in the middle of a woman's menstrual years does not mean that it cannot and does not occur early or late—in adolescence, or during and after menopause.

If endometriosis is caused by retrograde menstruation, which is the most common theory, it is unlikely that symptoms would appear for five years or so after menarche, thus making it illogical that a young adolescent would have it. But they do, so there must be other contributory factors:

- If the disease is hereditary, or at least has a strong familial tendency, it would make sense for symptoms to appear when menstruation begins because the girl would already have the disease.

- If endometrial tissue has migrated, it could begin to cause symptoms even before the hormonal system is fully functional.

- If endometriosis is caused by autoimmunity, hormonal influences are less relevant.

Teenagers who suffer from undue pain and other discomfort during menstruation should be taken to a gynecologist so that the endometriosis—if that's what it is—can be detected and treated early.

A gynecological examination can be painfully stressful and embarrassing for a young girl—far worse than it is for adults. For this reason, her mother should tell her *everything* that will happen. It'll sound pretty grim to a sensitive adolescent, but a mother who treats the experience as just another of the many unpleasant things that we have to do in our lives will be doing her daughter a favor. If she says, "Look, this exam is definitely not a day at the beach, but neither is it the worst thing in the world. Keep your mind calm, try to relax, and we'll go out and have a hot fudge sundae afterwards to celebrate getting through it," she will be encouraging her daughter to become an adult who takes responsibility for her own health.

But if she describes a trip to the gynecologist as horrible, painful, embarrassing, and ghastly in every imaginable way, she is setting her daughter up for a lifetime of fearful and hostile relationships with OBGs, and perhaps with doctors in general. Such an attitude is not conducive to preventive health care and good physical habits. It's also not very mature. Not only should you accompany your daughter to the gynecologist's office, you should go into the examining room with her and stay for the whole time. Hold her hand, stroke her forehead, talk to her sweetly, and let her know how brave she is being.

Although laparoscopy is the ultimate diagnosis for endometriosis, it is almost never necessary to subject young girls to this surgical procedure. The doctor will usually prescribe analgesics or nonsteroidal anti-inflammatory agents, which usually work well. If they don't, the doctor may start your daughter on oral contraceptives, which means that you need to have a heart-to-heart chat about the meaning of birth control and sexual activity. If none of these work, more drastic treatment might be required. See chapter 4 for a full discussion of treatment options.

Older Women

Older women, around age 45 and over, either premenopausal or postmenopausal, may have a condition known as *adenomyosis*, which is often confused with endometriosis. Adenomyosis involves endometrial tissue growing where it should not, but instead of being located outside the uterus, adenomyosis occurs inside the uterine muscle. It happens most frequently to women who have borne children, because the more children a woman has had, the weaker the uterine muscle and the more susceptible it is to invasion by endometrial tissue.

Endometriosis and adenomyosis usually don't coexist. If you had the former when you were younger, you probably will not have the latter when you're older. Adenomyosis is difficult to diagnose because, short of surgery, your doctor can't see the inside of your uterus. The organ can be palpated on manual examination, and it will feel enlarged and hard. It may also hurt when the doctor palpates it. There is no treatment for adenomyosis because it does not respond to hormonal therapy. And because it can sometimes be precancerous, most gynecologists recommend hysterectomy.

The presence of endometriosis itself after menopause, or before menopause when estrogen levels are diminishing, seems a contradiction. The apparent mechanism that brings on late endometriosis is the influence of extra-ovarian estrogen, that is, estrogen produced outside the ovaries. Surprise! You didn't know that happened. As menopause approaches, the adrenal glands convert fat cells (where estrogen is stored) into a weak form of estrogen called *estrone*, which produces some of the same effects as ovarian estrogen. And because estrogen is stored in fat cells, the more overweight you are, the longer your endometriosis will hang around. Nonsurgical treatment for menopausal endometriosis is the same as it is for younger women, but drug dosages are adjusted accordingly.

Accompanying Problems

As if endometriosis weren't enough of a burden all by itself, it is sometimes accompanied by other problems:

- In March 1977, Swedish researchers reported on an analysis of more than 20,000 women hospitalized for endometriosis. They had a 20 percent greater risk of cancer (breast, ovary, blood, and especially non-Hodgkin's lymphoma) than women who did not have the disease. The researchers speculated that hormonal treatment of endometriosis increases cancer risk (Brinton, Gridley, et al., 1997).

- Women with endometriosis are twice as likely to get vaginal *Candida albicans* infection. The reason is unclear, but the most likely culprit is a possibly compromised immune system.

Prevention of Endometriosis: Is It Possible?

Some people believe that endometriosis might be prevented, or at least discouraged. Others think it is impossible to prevent a disease for which a cause is unknown. But if prevention is indeed possible, the steps one might take would depend on the causation theory, and remember that such a theory is nothing more than a reasonable hypothesis about something that has yet to be proved. However, if a woman has a strong hereditary history of endometriosis, nothing much can be done to prevent the disease. Theories of prevention are outlined below, but bear in mind that none of them, when put into practice, will absolutely counteract the disease:

- If anatomic abnormalities that result in reflux menstruation or that prevent menstrual fluid from flowing out of the body are corrected, the risk of endometriosis is decreased. This should be done before a woman reaches menarche. However, it is highly unlikely that many parents would subject a young girl to a comprehensive pelvic examination—let alone, major surgery in order to prevent a disease that may or may not occur.

- If a young woman begins using low-dose oral contraceptives as soon as she reaches menarche and continues using them regularly, growth of the endometrium will be limited and the amount of the menstrual flow reduced, thus lessening the risk of endometriosis. This has its drawbacks, too. How many parents are willing to give an eleven-, twelve- or thirteen-year-old birth control pills before she is sexually active? Also, no one knows what negative consequences will result from giving hormones to such young girls.

- Manipulative surgical and nonsurgical procedures should be avoided immediately before and during menstruation in order to prevent reflux menstruation. These procedures include tubal insufflation, vigorous pelvic examination, cryotherapy, cervical cauterization, conization of the cervix, procedures that abrade the vagina, removal of fibroid tumors or other surgery in which the uterus is punctured, and plastic surgery.

- It has been said that regular strenuous exercise, begun at an early age, reduces estrogen levels and leads to lighter and less painful menstrual periods. This protective influence may decrease the risk of endometriosis.

- There is a theory that delayed childbirth increases the risk of endometriosis because it creates long uninterrupted periods of hormonal cycling and it increases opportunity for seeding the pelvic cavity with displaced endometrial tissue. This implies that early pregnancy and childbirth would decrease the risk of the disease. There is, however, no scientific basis for this belief, and it is *not* a good reason to become pregnant before one is ready.

Whether endometriosis is preventable remains to be seen; women will either get it or they won't. There are two important things to remember, however. If you or your daughter gets it, it's not your or her fault. There is most likely nothing you could have done to prevent it, so there's no reason to feel guilty. Second, if and when the disease does occur, get it diagnosed and treated as quickly as possible. As with all diseases, the earlier the treatment, the less painful and complicated it will be.

3

Pain

Endometrial lesions don't always hurt. In fact, some women don't know they have the disease because they have never experienced pain. Most, however, have at least some pain at least some of the time.

One of the more frustrating things about endometriosis is that there is no correlation between the severity of the disease, as measured by the number, size, and location of lesions, and the intensity and frequency of pain. However, some research has shown that there may be a correlation between depth of infiltration of lesions, that is, how deeply they are imbedded into the tissue where they have settled, and intensity of pain.

The pain associated with endometriosis often includes ordinary menstrual cramps as well as the low back pain that many women experience with their periods. Pain is caused by a number of other factors as well:

- Pain receptors in the cells of endometriomata are stretched or compressed, especially during menstruation.

- Endometrial cells release inflammatory chemicals such as prostaglandins and histamines.

- If cysts rupture, they too release these chemicals.

- When endometrial lesions invade tissues or organs such as the intestines or urinary bladder, they cause pain. If they leak blood, they will cause irritation and pain.

- Scar tissue and adhesions block or restrict access to blood vessels and deprive pain receptors of oxygen, a vital ingredient of normal cell function.

- A retroverted uterus or ovaries that adhere to the cul-de-sac may cause pain due to compression of the structures.

The pain of endometriosis is bad enough, but what is even worse, according to many women, is the fact that their doctors trivialize it, ignore it, refuse to believe it is as bad as it is, and utter those dreaded words, "It's all in your head." In many respects, the pain of endometriosis is regarded in a way that the pain of menstruation used to be: as a myth, as the price we pay for being women, or as an excuse to be cranky and out of sorts once a month. Few people believed that things were all that bad when women doubled over and went to bed with a hot water bottle for a day or two each month. Then research showed that menstrual pain was real, that there is a biochemical basis for it (prostaglandins cause uterine contractions, which can be quite strong), and that it can be treated. Menstruation and its difficulties "came out of the closet" and turned up as a real subject to be researched by serious scientists. Researchers at pharmaceutical companies discovered that two major classes of drugs can relieve menstrual cramps: prostaglandin synthetase inhibitors and nonsteroidal anti-inflammatory drugs (NSAIDs).

As often happens in medical research, once a symptom or other event can be explained and measured, it becomes "real" and the search for treatment follows. This is beginning to happen in endometriosis, but unfortunately too many physicians, including OBGs who should know better, aren't yet prepared to take your pain seriously. If your doctor is like that, find another one (more about how to do that in chapter 7).

The Mystery of Endometriosis Pain

There are a number of puzzling aspects about the pain of endometriosis. Lack of correlation between severity of disease and intensity of pain remains a mystery. Some think that painless disease may be biochemically inactive and less likely to release inflammatory substances, but this is only a theory. Some women's pain disappears spontaneously, perhaps because, although the lesions are still present, they have become less metabolically active. After many pain-free months, the endometriosis hurts again, and this cycle of waxing and waning pain may go on for years—or all the way to menopause. No one knows why it happens.

Laurel had excruciating pain right from the moment she began to menstruate. She feels fine now because the combination of surgical treatment and medication worked, but she frowned unconsciously as she talked about the pain. "My doctor, when I finally found one who took me seriously and was willing to do a laparoscopy, said I had a really teeny amount of endometriosis, but the pain was just unbelievable." She said that before surgery, she felt "at the end of my rope."

Some women still have pain even after all lesions have been surgically removed. This is another mystery. It may be that some lesions remain after surgery, and the disease is still present in a microscopic form. In addition, surgical adhesions can masquerade as endometrial pain, and there are probably ways in which endometriosis causes pain that are not yet understood.

Hysterectomy sometimes cures pain and sometimes does not. If most or all of the lesions were on the outside of the uterus, removing it will "cure" the disease. If there are lesions elsewhere, in addition to those on the uterus, hysterectomy will be somewhat but not totally effective. Some women also have phantom pain after removal of the uterus, just as people have phantom pain after amputation of a limb. There also is some speculation that endometriosis may create various disturbances in the immune system that results in dysfunction in pain receptors, or with coding and transmitting of pain signals along neural pathways.

Factors other than the presence of endometriomata may cause pain, for example a high level of inflammation in the pelvis. This is not as unusual as it seems. Other diseases and conditions cause pain without the person having "anything to show for it." For instance, a tension headache can be excruciating, but nothing would show up on an X ray or CAT scan done while the headache is in full force. Whiplash injury to the neck is another such example. Nothings shows on the X ray, but the pain can be severe, and analgesics, along with a neck brace and time to heal, usually work wonders. There is no reason why the same cannot be true for endometriosis, and regardless of what medical researchers discover in the future, you hurt now and you need relief.

This brings us to another subject: describing and locating the pain. It's never easy for most of us to put feelings into words, and when it comes to pain, many find it even more difficult. A good physician will want a highly detailed description of the character and severity of the pain, and fumbling for the words to describe it while you're sitting in the doctor's office puts you in an awkward position. So as soon as you make the appointment, start thinking about your pain and make notes about it. The following list outlines what the doctor will want to know and what you will need to describe:

- the character of the pain, that is, what it feels like: dull, throbbing, stabbing, burning

- the exact location

- when it begins, how long it lasts, and whether the severity increases with each bout of pain

- what you have done to relieve the pain and whether and how well your efforts work

- other symptoms that accompany the pain such as headache, dizziness, nausea and/or vomiting, excessive menstrual flow, diarrhea, or constipation

- whether bouts of pain have a relationship to anything else such as eating, exercising, sexual activity, or increased stress

Keep a diary of your pain and other symptoms and be sure to record all the drugs you take.

Pain Management

Medications

There are a number of ways to alleviate pain, the best of which is with analgesic drugs (*analgesia* means pain relief). Many women shy away from drugs because they prefer not to take pills and think that analgesics will do them more harm than the endometriosis. This is not true if you take the drugs according to directions. Read the label of any drug you take, prescription or over the counter, and don't exceed the recommended dose. If you follow these guidelines, you should be fine.

NSAIDs are widely prescribed for the pain of menstruation as well as that of endometriosis. These drugs work by interfering with pain signals that travel along peripheral pathways. Many NSAIDs can be purchased over the counter, although the strength is usually half that of the prescription counterpart. These drugs do not all act in the same way; they provide higher and lower levels of analgesia and anti-inflammatory action. The best way to find out which one works best for you is by trial and error. Commonly available NSAIDs include:

- naproxen sodium (its prescription names are Anaprox and Naprosyn; its over-the-counter name is Aleve)

- ketorolac tromethamine (Toradol)

- indomethacin (Indocin)

- ibuprofen (its most widely known over-the-counter names are Motrin and Advil)

Some people experience gastrointestinal distress with NSAIDs, but a change in drug usually makes the problem go away. The best way to take NSAIDs is before the pain gets too severe. In other words, don't wait until you're in agony to take the pill(s).

The NSAID that most women take for endometriosis pain is Motrin. In fact, every woman interviewed for this book described positive experiences with the drug. Lorraine said, "My life changed completely when I discovered Motrin in high school." Dulcie "discovered" Motrin when she was a student nurse and learned how to adjust doses according to the amount of pain she was having.

Narcotics, also called opiates, are highly effective analgesics, but they have serious side effects: drowsiness, constipation, and respiratory depression. These drugs (such as morphine, codeine, and Demerol) act on the central nervous system (the brain and spinal cord) to dull the perception of pain. In other words, what hurts you still hurts, you just aren't aware of it. The drugs are extremely addictive and should be used only when everything else has failed. Some doctors prescribe a small dose of a narcotic combined with a small dose of an NSAID because they find this often works well. The process is known to doctors as potentiation and to the rest of us as "piggybacking."

Some women find pain relief with over-the-counter topical creams or gels rubbed into the skin. Capsicum ointment (Zostrix or Capsagel) made from pulverized hot pepper seeds can improve circulation and relieve pain by increasing production of endorphins (naturally occurring chemicals that diminish pain). Topical lidocaine (Emla) also works sometimes by freezing adjacent tissues. These topical agents are available without a prescription, and again, the best approach is to try various remedies.

Aspirin and other salicylates as well as acetaminophen (Tylenol) work well for pain, although some women find that they need to take higher and higher doses. If this happens, you should switch to an NSAID on the advice of your physician. Aspirin also can cause gastric irritation and other gastrointestinal upsets. If this is a problem for you, buy coated tablets or aspirin buffered with a substance that counteracts its acid (Bufferin is a commonly found product). Aspirin can interfere with blood clotting, and high doses of acetaminophen can cause anemia and liver or kidney damage. If you do not exceed the recommended dose, you should be all right, but if you take more than the recommended dose and are worried about your liver or kidneys, your physician can check them with a blood test.

Chronic pain almost always results in stress, anxiety, and depression, and many women find themselves walking out of the doctor's office with a prescription for a tranquilizer or antidepressant. This may be appropriate in certain circumstances, but these drugs do not relieve pain and they certainly don't address the underlying problem of endometriosis. So, unless you have psychiatric problems (in which case you should be seeing a psychotherapist as well as an OBG), you would do better to treat the endometriosis rather than the anxiety and depression it causes.

Be aware that those physicians who hand out psychotropic drugs for physical problems are sending you a tacit message that you should not have to hear: "I don't believe there's anything wrong with you, but I don't want to lose you as a patient"; "There's probably something wrong with you, but I don't know how to diagnose it, so I'll try to make you feel better with tranquilizers"; "I can't stand listening to women like you complain, and these drugs are a good way to keep you quiet."

This indictment of OBGs and other physicians may sound harsh, but unfortunately it is often the reality of how many of them practice medicine. There is a lot of incompetence out there in the world in general, and the world of medicine is no different. In chapters 6 and 7, we'll talk about how to find and keep a good doctor—and how to recognize a inept doctor when you find yourself sitting across the desk from one.

Drug-free Pain Management

Drugs are not your only recourse in the management of the pain of endometriosis. Other methods include:

- Acupuncture (see chapter 8). This can be highly effective, but it doesn't work for everyone.

- Acupressure. Based on the same theoretical principles as acupuncture, this technique uses pressure instead of needles.

- Electrotherapy (transcutaneous electrical nerve stimulation). Electrotherapy doesn't always work, but when it does, pain relief is so fast that it seems miraculous. A small battery powered machine conducts an alternating current through electrode pads placed on the area that hurts or on nerve networks that control those areas.

- Heat. In the form of a hot bath, shower, whirlpool, or sauna, heat often relieves pain. It's also relaxing. Hot compresses or a heating pad work well too, but be careful not to burn yourself. If you have a cat who will lie quietly for a while, lie down with it on your belly. The cat's body heat works as well as an electrical pad, and the purring is relaxing.

- Massage. This soothing technique relieves muscle tension, which decreases pain.

- Shiatsu. This is a Japanese finger pressure technique that is similar to the Chinese acupressure and works on the same principles.

- Correcting your posture. Your mother was right when she told you to stand up straight, because improved posture often relieves abdominal pain.

- Moderate exercise. Swimming, walking, and bicycling can relieve pain and reduces stress.

- Weight loss. If you are overweight, try to shed a few pounds. Excess fatty tissue can put stress on pelvic and abdominal organs and thus increases pressure on endometriomata.

- Biofeedback. This approach might help (see chapter 8).

- Guided imagery. Also known as active imagination and visualization, guided imagery helps you create pain-free images for yourself while you are in a trance-like state. These images serve as a mental stimulus that "competes" with the pain or moves the pain to a less bothersome location. Guided imagery takes a while to learn, but if you can find a practitioner who can lead you through the process, it may be worth the effort.

- Hypnosis. This works for some people, as does self-hypnosis (see chapter 8).

- Relaxation. There are well-designed relaxation programs on tape that might be useful. Check out a few from the library before you invest your money in purchasing them.

Consequences of Chronic Pain

The consequences of severe and/or chronic pain are devastating and can wreak havoc with your entire life. Anxiety and stress have a deleterious effect. This is especially true in endometriosis because you never know when the pain will attack and how bad it will be. Some women are so emotionally crippled by anxiety and stress that they hesitate to make plans, because past experience has taught them that pain can be severe enough to require canceling activities. This is terrible for your social and professional life, and it quickly becomes intolerable. Moreover, anxiety and stress intensify pain so the whole syndrome turns into a vicious cycle.

Behavior modification and/or psychotherapy is probably indicated when things have reached this point.

Depression that can result from continued pain and anxiety is a serious psychological disorder. It needs to be treated before it gets so bad that you can't function. Symptoms of depression include apathy, inertia, lethargy, appetite changes, changes in sexual desire, crying for no apparent reason, fatigue, guilt, feelings of hopelessness and helplessness, inability to concentrate, passivity, pessimism, and suicidal thoughts and attempts.

Many women with chronic pain say they feel out of control, as if their bodies are being taken over by forces they cannot control and do not understand. Other women surrender to invalidism and make the pain of endometriosis the center of their lives. They think of themselves as sick people, making a "career" out of the sick role, and they encourage family and friends to do the same. This does not lead to healthy relationships, or positive self-esteem, and marriages and close friendships have foundered as a result.

Some women feel stigmatized by chronic pain. They say that they feel as handicapped as someone on crutches or in a wheelchair, but people don't take their handicap seriously. If an illness or injury doesn't show, it doesn't exist—that's the attitude that many people with chronic pain have to put up with. People who suffer from such pain face a dilemma: if they complain about it, they're branded whiners or malingerers, and their friends and family soon lose patience. But if they make an effort to suffer in silence and keep a stiff upper lip, the pain is discounted as "not really as bad as you made us think it is." It's a no-win situation, and there is not much they can do about it except go quietly about their way of seeking relief.

A few of the following tips might not relieve your pain, but they may make you feel better about yourself:

- If your physician trivializes your pain or flat-out doesn't believe you, leave the care of that physician.

- If your friends act the same way, make certain you express your anger and hurt at their insensitive attitude. If they continue, reevaluate the friendship.

- Do something about your pain. There is no reason to suffer needlessly.

- Don't blame yourself for the pain (others will heap more than enough blame on you). After all, you didn't give yourself endometriosis and you didn't make it hurt so much.

- Try hard not to lose your sense of humor.

If you find yourself in one or more of these situations, you *must* do something about it. If none of the techniques described above is effective, consider asking your physician for a referral to a pain management specialist or a pain control clinic. Most physicians who specialize in pain control or management are neurologists. They usually work in medical centers, so if you don't live near a metropolitan area, you may have to travel a ways. But it's worth the time and effort if you can get your life back in order.

Pain control is a subspecialty of neurology, and the details are not within the scope of this book. Suffice it to say, though, that you will be put through a comprehensive battery of tests, such as: thermography (mapping your body's surface temperature), spinogram (testing the involvement of spinal pain pathways), nerve blocks (injections to identify nerves or nerve bundles involved in your pain), and other neurological assessments. There will surely be X rays and perhaps a CAT scan (computerized tomography) or an MRI (magnetic resonance imaging).

If you want to find a pain clinic, ask your doctor for a referral. If the doctor pooh-poohs the idea, ask your friends if they have heard of a good one. You'll be surprised at how many times you hear something like: "Oh, my friend Janie's husband was in agony and he found this place up in Baltimore that he swears by. He's a new man now that he's not in pain all the time."

If that doesn't work, call the local medical society, or look in the yellow pages under physicians. If you decide to take the latter route, make certain that the pain clinic is associated with a reputable hospital. Avoid free-standing independent pain clinics. They may be fine, but they also may be operated by quacks who will take your money and leave you in the same pain as they found you. If the pain clinic refuses to deal with your health insurance company, or if it requires cash up front, make a speedy exit. You also can try calling the American Chronic Pain Association in Rocklin, California at (916) 632-0922 or the National Chronic Pain Outreach Association in Manassas, Virginia at (703) 368-8844.

4

Treatment

Although endometriosis can't be cured in the sense that a bacterial infection can be cured with a course of antibiotics, or appendicitis can be cured with an operation, there are a number of highly effective treatments. Many of them work for a while and a surprising number continue to keep symptoms in abeyance for a long period of time.

Whatever your doctor suggests as a first line of treatment may not do much, but the second or third treatment attempt will probably do the trick. There is such a variety of things to try that sooner or later, you will get relief. This is good news.

Pregnancy as a "Cure" for Endometriosis

The bad news is that even in the late 1990s, when one would think that physicians would know better, pregnancy is still touted as a "cure" for endometriosis. This happened to Kathleen. She began menstruating when she was fourteen and almost immediately began having cramps with her periods. "They weren't disabling, and I didn't have them every month," she said. "But I seemed to suffer more than the other girls in high school."

During the summer between high school and college, Kathleen had sex for the first time. "I loved it and my boyfriend and I did it *all the time*." In addition to the pleasure of her first sexual experience, Kathleen found that her menstrual cramps all but disappeared that summer. Then she went off to college and the boyfriend did not, and for the first few months, until she found another boyfriend, she was chaste—and in pain almost every month.

Kathleen got married when she was in graduate school, and her gynecologist told her that if she were to become pregnant, her menstrual cramps would disappear. The word *endometriosis* was never mentioned, and in fact, Kathleen didn't know she had the disease until she had surgery several years later.

"But it seemed like a really bizarre thing to say," she said. "First of all, I'd been married less than a year and although I wanted children eventually, neither Kevin nor I was ready, and our marriage wasn't ready. Besides," she added, laughing in hindsight at the stupidity of it, "did the doctor think I was going to be pregnant forever? He never bothered to tell me what would happen after I had the baby."

Kathleen is smart and sophisticated, and even more than twenty years ago, she knew enough not to take such bad "medical" advice.

Jean didn't take the advice to become pregnant either. "I never really wanted children all that much in the first place," she said. "And by the time my endometriosis was diagnosed, my husband and I were in the process of breaking up, so it was a bad idea altogether." But still, she resented the fact that a doctor had told her to get pregnant.

Pregnancy and occasionally lactation, neither of which are medical interventions, will likely arrest endometriosis temporarily. But it always comes back, often with increased vengeance, after delivery. Even though the medical literature is filled with anecdotes about pregnancy not being a good way to treat endometriosis, OBGs persist in recommending it. This is irresponsible.

An effort to get rid of endometriosis is not a morally, emotionally, or socially good reason to become pregnant—the most important decision a woman will ever make. Moreover, endometriosis is almost as unpredictable during pregnancy as it is in the nonpregnant state, and the disease occasionally has been known to get worse during pregnancy.

There are other reasons not to "treat" endometriosis with pregnancy:

- The disease increases the risk of ectopic pregnancy, which is a serious, life-threatening condition.

- Many women for whom pregnancy is recommended as a treatment are ill-equipped and ill-prepared to have a baby, or they just don't want one. But they feel vulnerable and powerless because of the ravages of the disease and thus make an unwise decision.

- The longer one has endometriosis, the greater the risk of infertility. Therefore, some women, in an attempt to "beat the clock," become pregnant before they really want to and before they are ready to—another unwise decision.

- Pregnancy should not be "prescribed" by a physician or suggested by anyone other than the woman herself and her husband or life partner. To do so, even in the guise of being helpful, is arrogant and highly unprofessional.

Types of Treatment

In terms of "real" treatment for endometriosis, no one actually knows what is the best thing to do, because no one fully understands what causes the disease. There is no absolute cure, and because of the variety and severity of symptoms, treatment is generally aimed at removing or shrinking endometriomata and restoring normal pelvic anatomy. Even so, the disease returns in about half the patients after two or three years of "successful" treatment, at which time another treatment should be tried.

There are three general approaches to treatment: medical, surgical, and a combination of both.

Medications

Hormonal Drug Therapy

Hormonal drugs stop ovulation and force endometriosis into remission. This occurs during the actual treatment and sometimes for years afterward.

Giving *progesterone* alone works by inhibiting the effect of estrogen on endometrial tissue, thus shrinking it. This is thought to be due to the effect of progesterone on the estrogen receptors of the endometrium. Treatment with progesterone does not appear to improve fertility.

Types of progesterones include:

- Those chemically derived from natural progesterone such as medroxyprogesterone acetate (brand names Amen, Cycrin, Provera) and progestin. Medroxyprogesterone acetate is taken at a dose of 10–50 mg a day by mouth for six to nine months. It also can be given by injection every two weeks.

- Derivatives of male hormones such as norethindrone (Aygestin) and norgestrel. Norethindrone is taken at a dose of 2.5–10 mg a day by mouth.

Side effects of these drugs vary depending on dosage, treatment interval, and route of administration. They include transient breakthrough bleeding, nausea, breast tenderness, fluid retention, and depression.

Progesterone treatment should be taken by women who have had all the children they want, because the drugs suppress ovarian function. It can take a year or more to recover this function.

A *combination of estrogen and progesterone*, like that found in oral contraceptives, is often called the pseudopregnancy regimen; it is the most commonly prescribed treatment for endometriosis, even though there is little scientific data about its efficacy. The anecdotal evidence is another story, however, because women say that the symptoms of the disease improve with combination therapy. It also shrinks endometrial tissue. But in studies with rhesus monkeys, some animals had even larger endometrial implants after combination therapy, which conflicts with the belief about its effect in humans (Damewood, Kresch, and Metzger, 1997). In reality, no one understands the effects of combination therapy on fertility or on the disease itself. It is typical of the trial-and-error approach to treating endometriosis.

Oral combination hormones, which can be administered either orally or by injection, include:

- norethynodrel and mestranol

- norethindrone acetate and ethanol estradiol

- lynestrol and mestranol

- morgestrel and ethanol estradiol

- 17-hydroxyprogesterone and Depo-Provera with stilbes-terol or Premarin as injectable forms of the therapy

Depending on the types of drugs given, side effects include nausea, high blood pressure, blood clots, enlargement of the uterus, acne, hair loss, increased muscle mass, decreased breast size, and deepening of the voice. If this list of side effects makes you pause, take heart. You won't turn into a man, but on the other hand, you need to think carefully about whether you are willing to tolerate some of these somewhat masculinizing effects.

Lorraine was given oral contraceptives in high school. Looking back, she knew she had endometriosis at the time, but it hadn't been definitively diagnosed. "I was put on birth control pills because they were supposed to help menstrual cramps, and they did, to an extent," she said. "But I got all these lectures about sexual promiscuity, from the doctor, from my mother, from just about everyone it seemed."

Lorraine went to high school in the late 1960s when the women's movement was just getting into full swing. "But even so, we never talked about periods and stuff like that, and no one else I knew took birth control pills. You weren't supposed to make a big deal about your period, and you weren't supposed to let it put you in bed for two or three days every month."

So Lorraine suffered in silence. Some months the oral contraceptives worked at controlling the pain, and some months they didn't. When they didn't, she took codeine, a narcotic analgesic that is probably not an appropriate drug for an adolescent. When she got to college, she discovered Motrin, which she said was the best thing that had happened to her thus far in terms of controlling the pain.

Except for the time she was trying to get pregnant, Lorraine has been on and off oral contraceptives for thirty years. Now, at age forty-five, she has taken Loestrin (a combination of norethindrone acetate and ethinyl estradiol) every day for the past two years. "I've never felt better in my life."

When Linda was fifteen and had been suffering from endometriosis since she began to menstruate, her mother took her to a gynecologist who put her on oral contraceptives. Did the doctor diagnose the endometriosis? "No, the word was never mentioned, and I still didn't know what was wrong with me. The doctor said that birth control pills often calmed down cramps."

Did they? "Yeah, they worked pretty well. I still had some pain sometimes with my periods, but nothing like what it had been. I really felt a lot better."

Linda took the pills for four years, and then all of a sudden, she started reacting badly to them. "A few hours after I took the pill, I would get sick, retching and throwing up. At first, I thought there was something else wrong with me, but then I read the label on the package, and it said that nausea and vomiting were a side effect. That went on for about two months, and I decided to stop taking them." She discussed it with her doctor who offered a substitute: Depo-Provera by injection once a month. That worked pretty well before her endoscopic surgery.

Gestrinone, an anti-progestational steroid, is used widely in Europe and South America. It is believed to decrease estrogen and progesterone receptors in the normal endometrium, but it is not known whether gestrinone has the same action in the presence of endometriosis. However, it may inhibit production of ovarian hormones, which is one of the goals of endometriosis treatment.

Gestrinone has been effective in alleviating pain and reducing the number and size of endometriomata. There is no evidence that it enhances fertility. Most side effects are usually mild and transient, but others, including voice changes, development of facial hair, and enlargement of the clitoris, can be permanent. A dose of 2.5 mg twice a week can significantly reduce the number of endometriomata in mild to moderate disease.

Mifepristone (better known as RU486) is the controversial abortifacient (an agent that induces abortion). It inhibits ovulation and disrupts the normal anatomy and physiology of the endometrium. Mifepristone's ability to cause regression of endometrial lesions varies depending on the duration of treatment. There is no evidence about its effect on pain. Side effects include hot flashes, fatigue, nausea, and changes in liver function.

Gonadotropin-releasing hormone (GnRH) agonists, such as goserelin acetate (Zoladex), given in a dose of 3.6 mg once a month as a subcutaneous injection, nafarelin acetate (Synarel), taken in two 200 mcg doses a day as a nasal spray, and leuprolide acetate (Lupron), given at a dose of 3.75 mg once a month as an intramuscular injection, have been highly effective against the pain of endometriosis. A transdermal patch will likely be on the market soon.

GnRH agonists also are used in other gynecologic disorders such as fibroid tumors, premenstrual syndrome, polycystic ovarian disease, and heavy menstrual bleeding. GnRH agonists work by first overloading and then desensitizing the pituitary gland, which secretes important sex hormones. In a two-step process, the drugs stimulate the ovaries to produce more than normal estriol (one of the several types of estrogen). After two to three weeks of constant stimulation, the pituitary ceases production of hormones that control the ovaries, which causes the ovaries to cease functioning. This pseudomenopausal state shrinks endometrial tissue. The treatment is sometimes known as medical oophorectomy because the ovaries are hormonally shut down without having to be surgically removed.

The advantages of GnRH agonists are that they have fewer and less severe side effects than other hormonal drugs, especially danazol, and ovulation and menstruation return quickly after the drug is discontinued.

There are two major disadvantages of GnRH agonists. First, they do not cure endometriosis; rather, they put it into temporary remission. Second, minor loss of bone density (3–5%) has been noted (Edmonds, 1996). The bone loss is reversible when the drug is withdrawn, but the side effect is of greatest concern when GnRH agonist treatment continues for more than six months, or when it is given to women over age forty. To prevent bone loss, it is recommended (Edmonds, 1996) that prolonged courses of treatment be accompanied by low-dose estrogen-progesterone therapy.

Add-back hormone replacement therapy can alleviate the hypoestrogenic (low levels of estrogen) effects of GnRH agonists, including loss of bone mineral content. This presents a dilemma for women with endometriosis because reintroduction of estrogen could exacerbate the disease. However, studies (Edmonds, 1996) have shown that giving GnRH in combination with hormone replacement therapy, using very low doses of estrogen and continuous (rather than cyclical) medroxyprogesterone acetate, greatly diminishes loss of bone mineral density without reducing the efficacy of the GnRH agonist.

GnRH antagonists inhibit the release of gonadotropin and have an immediate effect. These drugs are still in the experimental stage and have been plagued by a high percentage of allergic responses.

Testosterone, a male hormone produced in small amounts in the ovaries, can reduce pelvic pain and painful intercourse, and it does not affect ovulation so fertility is not impaired. However, it cannot be used for relief of infertility.

Danazol, a synthetic androgen (brand names: Danocrine and Cyclomen), has become increasingly popular, and for some women, it is highly effective. It was the first drug approved by the Food and Drug Administration specifically for the treatment of endometriosis. It is very expensive and carries serious side effects, including weight gain, muscle cramps, hot flashes, mood changes, acne, loss of libido, headache, hot flashes, deepening of the voice, and increased hair growth. Some women who take high doses of danazol find that their menstrual periods stop.

In addition, danazol has a negative effect on blood lipids (fats). It decreases high-density lipoproteins (HDLs), the so-called "good" cholesterol, but very low-density lipoproteins are unchanged. There has been some concern about atherosclerosis (hardening of the arteries, a condition that can lead to heart attack and stroke), but all effects on lipoproteins are reversed three to five months after danazol therapy is discontinued. Women who are taking warfarin to prevent blood clot formation should *not* take danazol.

Danazol must be taken over a long period of time (at least six months), during which you should not become pregnant because of the strong possibility of abnormal fetal development (use an effective barrier method of contraception such as a diaphragm or a high-quality condom).

The drug works primarily by suppressing normal pituitary-estrogen signaling, which decreases production of estrogen. It also inhibits certain enzymes responsible for estrogen production in the adrenal glands and ovaries. However, there is no direct evidence that danazol affects endometrial lesions; therefore, it probably works as a result of overall lowered estrogen. It also decreases the inflammatory response to endometrial lesions, which helps alleviate pain. The usual dose is 400–800 mg twice a day by mouth for three to six months.

In general, danazol has the following effects on women with endometriosis:

- It can "cure" mild to moderate disease.

- Lower daily doses (less than 400 mg a day) appear to be as effective as higher doses for less severe disease.

- Ovarian endometriomata do not respond well to danazol.

- Individual response is highly variable.

- It reduces endometriosis-associated autoimmune abnormalities.

In several studies, "second look" laparoscopy (the first look refers to the original laparoscopic procedure done to diagnose endometriosis) has revealed significant improvement in endometriosis after danazol therapy (Matalliotakis, Neonaki, et al, 1997). The less severe the disease, the more improvement. In some cases, endometriosis was totally resolved. Treatment with danazol had no effect on adhesions, however, and some women still require surgery if the pain of adhesions is severe.

In terms of pain relief, danazol is effective in combating painful menstruation, usually within two months of the onset of treatment. But it is less effective in chronic pelvic pain, which may or may not result from endometriomata but arise instead from adhesions or scarring. It has the advantage of not causing bone loss that is usually associated with lowered levels of estrogen, and a few women on the drug have even gained bone mass.

Danazol's effect on fertility varies greatly. Although no studies have proven this to be true, many physicians think that the severity of the disease matters when assessing post-treatment fertility. In other words, the worse the endometriosis, the less likely that danazol will help fertility, perhaps because ovarian endometriomata are more common in severe disease.

After Kathleen's surgery when she was twenty-five years old, her doctor wanted her to get pregnant right away, or at least to go on hormone therapy for a year to stop ovarian function and "to make sure that little microscopic patches of endometrium didn't take hold and start growing."

He gave her a choice: pregnancy, birth control pills, or danazol, which was then a brand new drug. "I still wasn't ready to get pregnant," she said. "And I sure as hell wasn't going to have a baby as a prescription. Danazol had some pretty weird side effects. I didn't want my husband describing me as the one with the deep voice and the beard!"

Kathleen took oral contraceptives for a year during which she didn't menstruate at all. The first year she went off the pills, her periods were sporadic and the bleeding was much lighter than usual.

Now, at age twenty-one and less than a year after laparoscopic surgery, Linda says that she can feel the endometriosis symptoms returning, so she thinks she will go back on Depo-Provera. Has she given any thought to danazol? "Yes, but the side effects seem pretty awful. I really hate the idea of taking male hormones."

Jean took danazol for six months when she was thirty-one years old. She didn't "turn into a man," as she put it, but she did have definite side effects: her face broke out, her breasts shrank, she had terrible headaches, and she got very aggressive, "snarly all the time," as she put it. "But the worst thing," she said, grimacing at the memory, "was that although I didn't have my period the whole time, I had this constant brown, yucky discharge. It was disgusting, and a real drag on my sex life, so I stopped the danazol."

Hormone Replacement Therapy

All women who have had their ovaries removed surgically (bilateral oophorectomy), not just those with endometriosis, ought to give some thought to hormone replacement therapy (HRT). However, the decision to take replacement hormones is more difficult for women with endometriosis because taking estrogen after menopause (surgical or natural) has been known to make the disease recur. After going to all the trouble, pain, and expense of having your ovaries out in order to treat endometriosis, you might want to think twice about "daring" it to come back with hormones. Then again, the estrogen may have no adverse effects at all on your "former" disease. There is not enough evidence to know for certain what will happen.

A full discussion of HRT is not within the scope of this book. There are plenty of books with this information in the library and bookstores; what follows here is simply a general overview of the advantages and disadvantages of HRT.

Losing your ovaries also can mean losing your sex drive, or at least a good part of it. The medical term for this is loss of libido, and it is very common after oophorectomy. HRT can get your sexual urges revved up again. Depending on your age, the state of your love life, and your general feelings about sex, this may or may not be important to you.

There has been a good deal of controversy in the medical community in the last decade or so about the risk of cancer for women taking unopposed estrogen (estrogen alone without progesterone) as HRT. Those who suggest that there might be an increased risk of breast and endometrial cancers, stressed that the risk was statistically very low. However, when progesterone is added to estrogen on a cyclical basis, the risk of cancer is no greater than it would be naturally in women of postmenopausal age; that is, there is *no* increased risk. Therefore, it seems that, in terms of the risk of cancer anyway, you are in no danger from HRT.

Postmenopausal women are at increased risk of osteoporosis which is diminution of bone mass. Bones become lighter and more fragile, thus increasing the risk of fractures. There is a good deal of evidence to suggest that HRT has a positive effect on bone mass and can retard the progress of osteoporosis. It also seems to have a protective effect on the cardiovascular system.

You can take HRT in one of three general ways: by mouth, as a vaginal cream, and as a transdermal patch. Probably the most popular way to take HRT is a fairly new drug called Prempro. It is a combination of conjugated estrogens of the type found in the old standby Premarin and progesterone in the form of medroxyprogesterone acetate. You take one tablet a day, every day and that's all there is to it. There's nothing to count, no thinking about what day of the cycle you're at, and best of all, for the vast majority of women, there is no breakthrough bleeding. In other words, no more periods.

Vaginal creams are inserted into the vagina with an applicator. Although the hormone is absorbed into the bloodstream and thus affects other parts of the body, its major influence is on the vagina itself. This HRT route is probably best suited to women whose major menopausal symptoms center on her vagina and urethra (manifesting in more urinary tract infections).

The transdermal patch also is fairly new, and women either like it or they don't. The estrogen contained in the patch that you wear on your abdomen (and change once or twice a week) is absorbed directly into the bloodstream at a controlled rate, much like the patches that people wear when they are trying to quit smoking or trying not to throw up on an airplane. The advantage of taking HRT this way is that the drug bypasses the liver and digestive system, thus avoiding problems that can occur when the drug passes through these organs. And it's good for people who can't remember to take a pill every day (of course, you have to remember to change the patch). The disadvantages are that it can cause skin rash, and in hot, wet climates, it may not stick to your skin very well.

Hormonal Drug Side Effects

Many hormonal drug treatments, especially GnRH agonists and antagonists, have side effects in common, and those effects can be extremely annoying. Following are some suggestions for dealing with them:

- If you get hot flashes, wear loose cotton clothing, cut down on caffeine and alcohol, stay away from hot foods and liquids (hot in temperature as well as spice content) if you find they trigger hot flashes, drink lots of water, eat foods high in Vitamins C, A, and D, sleep with lighter-than-usual covers (in winter, substitute an electric blanket for a down comforter because the temperature is adjusted easily), and do moderate to strenuous exercise regularly.

- Vaginal dryness is easy to remedy with a water-soluble lubricant such as K-Y Jelly or Astro Glide. They are available in drugstores without a prescription. Make certain you don't use an oily lubricant such as Vaseline, olive oil, or baby oil. In addition, longer, more intense foreplay will allow your own natural lubricants to flow more easily. Above all, don't force yourself to have sex if you're not in the mood.

- If the treatments give you headaches, limit the amount of salt and salty foods you eat, and stay away from monosodium glutamate (MSG), both of which cause increased fluid retention, which can result in headaches. Many headaches are caused by constriction of blood vessels in the head. Foods made with yeast, alcohol, aged cheeses, and processed meats (lunch meat, hot dogs, and canned meat like Spam) sometimes cause blood vessel constriction.

- If you suffer from mood swings, you might want to find a support group and talk about it. You probably don't need "real" psychotherapy, but sharing your feelings and experiences with women who are going through what you are can be very helpful.

- Do whatever you can to reduce the stress in your life (see chapter 6).

Nonhormonal Drugs

Other medications used to treat endometriosis include:

- Gossypol, a drug widely used in China, has been shown to reduce estrogen levels and shrink endometriomata. It also provides pain relief. There is no evidence one way or the other about its effect on fertility, and it may have a toxic effect on the kidneys.

- Tamoxifen, an anti-estrogen, is used to treat breast and ovarian cancer, but because it is an estrogen antagonist and suppresses uterine growth, it may be effective in endometriosis. Only one very small study on the use of tamoxifen in endometriosis has been done so far, and the results were "iffy." (Damewood, Kresch, and Metzger, 1997) Pain decreased and endometriomata shrank while the women were on the drug but returned as soon as it was withdrawn. The women continued to ovulate, but none became pregnant while on tamoxifen. Side effects include hot flashes, fatigue, constipation, and acne, all of which disappeared within six months after stopping treatment.

Surgery

Surgery is often indicated in endometriosis. Treatment should begin with the most nonradical and least invasive procedures and proceed "upward" as the surgical procedures fail. The least radical surgery, that is, laparoscopy, appears to have the fewest long-term negative effects such as adhesions, which many physicians believe cause pain and infertility.

During any type of surgery for endometriosis, all tissue removed from your body should be sent to the laboratory for examination under a microscope (biopsy). This is done, not because it is likely that any of the tissue is malignant (it hardly ever is), but because something that looks like endometriosis may not be, and tissue that does not resemble an endometrial lesion might indeed be. Moreover, endometrial cysts are easily mistaken for something else, and vice versa.

Microscopic tissue examination is not something you really need to discuss with your doctor, unless you're the kind of person who wants to be aware of every detail, because all reputable hospitals have a regulation that *all* tissue removed in the operating room will be subjected to such examination—regardless of the tissue or type of surgery. It is a routine part of being a surgical patient, like having your blood drawn and giving a urine sample.

There is a good deal of controversy in the medical community about the success of surgery in endometriosis. Since it is *possible* to remove most, if not all, endometriomata, it is assumed that this constitutes successful treatment. However, once the operation is over, the patient is subject to the same pathologic processes that caused the disease in the first place, and there is no reason to prevent it from coming back full blast. In fact, it does in 25 to 50 percent of all women who were surgically treated.

There is also much debate about the effect of surgery on fertility. It's impossible to know if surgery will enhance fertility if you don't know if you're infertile to begin with. This in itself is difficult to determine. Moreover, disease severity affects both fertility and the success of surgery. That is, the worse the disease, the greater the likelihood of infertility and the less likely that surgery will be successful. The "answer" to the question of fertility, then, is that it's impossible to know if you will be able to get pregnant after surgery.

Laparoscopy

Laparoscopy is the least invasive procedure and is used to confirm the diagnosis, determine the extent of disease, and remove small endometrial deposits. It is the preferred method of surgical treatment, mainly because the physician can treat at the same time that diagnosis is made. In addition, you are under anesthesia for a relatively short time, your hospital stay is shorter (you usually don't have to stay overnight), and you recuperate faster than from more extensive surgery.

However, laparoscopy requires more technical skill and experience than more invasive operations, so women should be certain to ask their OBGs how long they have been doing the procedure and how many they average in a week.

As a treatment for endometriosis, rather than solely as a diagnostic tool, laparoscopy is effective only in mild to moderate cases.

The procedure consists of inserting a long, thin hollow tube into the abdominal cavity through a very small incision inside or close to the umbilicus. This tube is inserted after the abdomen has been distended with carbon dioxide gas (you will have severe gas pains for a day or two after your operation). A light attached to fiberoptic bundles is then threaded through the tube so the surgeon can see the inside of the abdomen. In addition to a light, various surgical tools also can be inserted through the tube to accomplish any of the following:

- Various mechanical procedures include grasping, pinching, and clamping diseased tissue.

- Electrosurgery uses electric current to deal with tissue by vaporization (destruction by instant boiling of intracellular water), coagulation (heating and drying tissue to kill it), and fulguration (superficial burning with a spark of electricity). There are two types of electrosurgery: unipolar in which the current passes through the body of the patient, and bipolar in which it passes through only the tissue being held by the surgical instrument. Electrosurgery is reasonably safe *if* it is done by an experienced surgeon. If your doctor proposes this procedure, ask about experience, that is, number of such procedures done in the past. The two biggest dangers in electrosurgery are inadvertently applying current to the wrong tissue (or burning through an endometrial lesion to the underlying structure), and fire in the operating room if live current accidentally comes in contact with surgical drapes, which are now made mostly of paper.

- Laser (an acronym for *l*ight *a*mplification by the *s*timulated *e*mission of *r*adiation) surgery has become so popular for so many ailments that many people feel cheated if they don't get a laser treatment. In endometriosis, this tightly concentrated, intense energy beam is aimed at endometriomata and cuts, vaporizes, and coagulates in one swift motion. Four main types of lasers are in common use today: CO_2, YAG, KTP, and KTP/YAG combination. Some OBGs think that laser treatment is effective for only very superficial lesions, which are not the ones that usually cause severe pain.

- A brand new technique is an ultrasound scalpel with very high frequency sound waves that destroys tissue. The ultrasonic scalpel generates little heat, but some say it is more likely to damage healthy tissue. Again, women should ask their surgeons how much experience they have had with this technique.

- A hysterosalpingogram is a procedure in which dye is flushed through the fallopian tubes to determine their patency.

After laparoscopy, some doctors will put their patients on oral contraceptives for a few weeks to reduce the likelihood of recurrence of the disease; others feel this isn't necessary. Unfortunately, as with many other aspects of endometriosis, there are no definitive studies to serve as guidance about post-laparoscopy therapy.

Linda had a laparoscopy when she was twenty years old. It was done almost as an emergency. "I had had terrible diarrhea for about eight weeks—I mean really, really bad: going six or seven times a day. I got all dehydrated and ended up in the emergency room a few times because I almost passed out.

"I lost about fifteen pounds and looked like I had anorexia. Everybody at work made fun of me because my clothes were just hanging on me and because I was always running to the bathroom. It was awful."

Linda usually drove herself to the emergency room where she was always refused pain medication. "They started to think I was some kind of drug addict because I always asked for something for the pain, but I never got it. They were all male doctors."

During this period, Linda had gone to her family doctor about the uncontrollable diarrhea, but he just told her to keep taking Immodium, an over-the-counter anti-diarrhea remedy, which wasn't helping. It never helped, no matter how many doses she took.

Two days before her laparoscopic surgery, Linda's father took her to the emergency room because she was so doubled over with cramps and so weakened by the diarrhea that she couldn't drive herself. This time, when she asked for something for the pain, her father backed her up and apparently applied some verbal force to the request. She got a shot of Demerol, a narcotic analgesic. "It was wonderful," said Linda. "I had no idea how easily the pain could be relieved and how much better I could feel after the shot."

As Linda was preparing to go home, a nurse spoke to her about the number of times Linda had shown up there for similar kinds of pain. "I think you have endometriosis," the nurse told me. "She also said I ought to get right to my gynecologist. So I did the very next day."

That was the first time anyone had mentioned the word "endometriosis" to Linda. The day after that, Linda had her laparoscopy. A friend accompanied Linda to the hospital, stayed with her until the operation was over, and then drove her home. "I wouldn't have been able to get through it without her," said Linda. "It hurt terribly when I woke up, and it seemed to take forever for me to get my strength back. I stayed in bed for two or three days, and then after that, I started to feel better. My doctor told me I had a really bad case of endometriosis; it was all over my bladder and bowels, and she cauterized a lot of the stuff that wasn't supposed to be there." Linda shuddered at the idea of her own flesh burning, but she also acknowledged that her diarrhea went away, and whatever she ate didn't run through her right away.

So, slowly she gained back all the weight she had lost, and now she looks the picture of health. But she says she feels the symptoms coming back. Will she have another laparoscopy? She makes a face at the thought. "The last time, I was weak and debilitated going into the surgery, and this time, I'd like to do it before things deteriorate so badly."

Jean didn't have a very good experience with laparscopy either. "Everyone says it's a real nothing operation. You get the impression that you can just sort of jump off the operating table and go back to work that afternoon." This has never been true about laparoscopy, but many doctors downplay the fact that it's a real operation in a real hospital with real anesthesia. Because the incision is smaller than in other types of surgery does not mean that it can be taken lightly.

Jean stayed home from work for a week even though she went home the day of the surgery and spent only that afternoon and evening in bed. "I just didn't feel right," she said. "The incision hurt, and it took me a while to get over the anesthesia."

That, however, is normal. It *is* surgery and it *will* hurt for a few days. Spending only a day and an evening in bed after having an operation is a minor price to pay if the treatment works. But the pain of endometriosis came back the next month. "That was a real bummer," said Jean. Having a highly touted surgical procedure fail in its purpose is very disappointing.

Limited Surgery

Limited surgery is done through a regular abdominal incision called a laparotomy. The purpose is to remove adhesions and endometriomata that are too big to be pulled through a laparoscope. At the same time, the surgeon may sever certain pelvic nerves in an effort to relieve pain (called a presacral neurectomy). This type of surgery may preserve fertility, although no one knows why because the relationship of infertility to endometriosis is not well understood. If the uterus is retroverted, fixed, or otherwise abnormally situated, repair of it and other pelvic structures may be therapeutic. In addition, removal of adhesions and appendectomy may help, although no one knows why.

Limited (conservative) surgery may provide better and more long-lasting pain relief than laparoscopy because the surgeon is apt to remove more endometrial lesions—simply because more of them are open to view with a larger incision. But recurrence rates are reported to be as high as 40 percent after limited surgery, so it's hard to say whether you will be better off with a bigger or smaller operation. This is just one more of the many frustrations of endometriosis: not knowing in advance what the likelihood of success will be.

Kathleen had a laparotomy for what she and her doctor thought was a large ovarian tumor. When she was twenty-five years old, her doctor found a lump on her left ovary. "I went back for an exam every two weeks because he wanted to watch it and see if it grew. It did.

"I had an ultrasound a few months later that showed a large cyst. By that time, it hurt even when he wasn't poking around inside me. The pain was especially bad when I walked upstairs and when I sat down."

The doctor recommended that it be removed, and Kathleen agreed. "I checked into the hospital the night before, and when I was given the consent form to sign, I was shocked. It said that I was giving permission for him to take out both ovaries, both tubes, and my uterus if he thought it was necessary.

"There was no way I was going to give permission for that much stuff. I was only twenty-five and I wanted children. So we agreed that the absolute most he could remove was my left ovary and fallopian tube. That way, I'd still have one to make babies with."

The operation went better than Kathleen had expected. "The cyst, which he said was the size of a grapefruit, peeled right off my ovary so I still have them both. It turned out to be a chocolate cyst, and that was the first time I knew I had endometriosis." This is not uncommon. Many women are not diagnosed until they have an operation.

So did the operation take care of the problem? "For about six months after surgery, I had some pain with my period, and that's when I started taking oral contraceptives. When I went off those, I had no pain at all. I started trying to get pregnant, and three years later, my daughter was born."

Kathleen has been symptom free for twenty years now.

Radical Surgery

Radical surgery, sometimes called complete hysterectomy, is removal of the uterus, both ovaries, and both fallopian tubes. Fertility is obviously destroyed as a result, but if a woman has all the children she wants (or if she does not want children), this may be the best approach because it is a highly effective treatment. But because it is so drastic, it should not be undertaken lightly.

Many women whose endometriosis is treated by removing their reproductive organs still suffer pain because endometrial lesions located on organs and structures other than the reproductive ones are still there. So if the surgeon does not remove all endometrial lesions at the time you have a complete hysterectomy, you might as well not have had an operation at all. This is unfortunate (actually, it's worse than unfortunate, it's a damn shame), but it happens all the time, so talk with your surgeon beforehand to find out exactly what's going to happen while you are under anesthesia.

Complete hysterectomy also results in what is called surgical menopause. It is essentially the same as natural menopause, but it happens suddenly and the woman is often psychologically unprepared for it, especially if she is younger than forty. Many women who undergo complete hysterectomy take hormone replacement therapy, which *may* cause a recurrence of endometriosis.

Other types of radical surgery include:

- removal of a ureter when endometriosis poses a serious threat to kidney function

- repair of a bowel obstruction or removal of a segment of the large bowel if the obstruction can't be repaired

- plastic surgery if the rectovaginal septum has deep endometrial implants

- removal of the uterus (usually with the fallopian tubes) because of severe endometrial involvement but with the ovaries left intact

Adhesions

We need to say a word or two here about *adhesions,* a postoperative phenomenon that can occur after any type of surgery but that seems particularly common after an operation to remove endometriomata.

Adhesions are bands of stretched scar tissue that bind together tissue surfaces, and sometimes organs, that are normally separate. They also can cause significant distortion of pelvic anatomy, which can be painful. Postoperative adhesions can cause as much pain and other trouble as did the original endometrial lesions. No one knows what causes adhesions to form so preventing them is a hit-or-miss situation. Various solutions and gels can be inserted into the operative site in an attempt to prevent tissue surfaces from adhering. Sometimes this works; sometimes it does not. Some people seem more prone to form adhesions, but there's no way to predict who will get them and who won't.

They are a major postoperative nuisance, and they are often extremely painful. In addition, depending on where the scar tissue is located, adhesions can cause large bowel obstructions. If adhesions pull the large bowel out of shape (the most common consequence), pain can be severe. They also cause bladder problems and impaired fertility.

If the adhesions are particularly large and significantly interfere with physiological function, complete surgical removal of the adhesion, not just cutting into it to ease the constriction, may be needed to remove them. This seems like a paradox: doing surgery to repair a condition that was caused by surgery in the first place. But a large or small bowel obstruction is agonizing and can be life threatening. If the adhesions cause only intermittent pain of moderate severity, it's probably best to do nothing or to experiment with nonsurgical treatment, such as Rolfing, deep muscle massage, and ultrasound therapy to alleviate the pain.

Many women just do nothing. Susan said, "Every three or four months, my belly hurts like hell. It almost always happens in the evening so I get into bed and wait for the pain to go away. It never lasts more than a few hours, and I can usually stand it without taking anything. If it's especially bad, I take three or four Advil or one of the prescription Tylenol with codeine that my dentist gave me after I had a tooth pulled. I let myself wallow in self-pity the whole time, and if the pain keeps me awake for part of the night, I call in sick the next day. But I'll be dammed if I'm going to have another operation!"

Coping with Hysterectomy

Until fifteen or twenty years ago, women dreaded the thought of a hysterectomy, because it signaled the end of reproductive life. This was a reasonable cause for grief and upset since many of us, at that time, believed that having children was our primary purpose in life.

But things are different now. Motherhood is only one facet of a woman's existence. Also, we have learned to take a greater interest in the way we allow doctors to treat us and in the way we think of ourselves. We don't let them whip out our uteruses at the drop of a hat or the first sign of a little heavier-than-normal menstrual flow. We ask questions; we want to know if a hysterectomy is *really* necessary, and what alternatives we should consider.

And when we really do have to have the operation, we don't fall apart when we hear the news. Surgery in general is easier now than it was twenty years ago. Anesthetic drugs are better, and postoperative routine gets patients up on their feet sooner than ever—in most cases, a few hours after they wake up. This prevents many postop complications. The incision is smaller so the postop pain is not as bad, and the scar it leaves is not as ugly and disfiguring. Nevertheless, hysterectomy *is* major surgery and you'll have to go into the hospital for it, so there are things you ought to know to be well prepared for the surgery and its aftermath.

When Helen had her hysterectomy, she didn't know she had endometriosis. At least she didn't know for certain. Both she and her gynecologic surgeon strongly suspected it. "I was told I needed a hysterectomy because I had a huge mass in my belly. It turned out to be a six pound fibroid. My doctor said it was like carrying around a six pound baby."

The size of the fibroid was probably an exaggeration (on the part of Helen or her doctor), but the extent of her endometriosis was not. Helen had had serious menstrual cramps every month of her life from the time she began menstruating at age eleven until the hysterectomy at age forty. Getting rid of her uterus and all the endometrial lesions must have been a relief.

"It was," Helen said. And she added that she hasn't suffered from those ghastly menstrual cramps. "But lately, every once in a while, I feel a little premenstrual twinge of something. It's not exactly pain, but it feels like I might be getting my period even though I'm not, because I don't have a uterus anymore."

Jean had a positive experience with hysterectomy. She had had a myomectomy (removal of a fibroid tumor) when she was forty, but of course that didn't do anything for the endometriosis. By the time she was forty-three, she was "swilling down some pretty serious pain pills [Toradol], and I just decided to be done with the whole thing and have my uterus out."

She had fairly radical surgery (one ovary was left in), but she feels fine now. The endometriosis is gone, and she has never felt better in her life. "My sex life is all shot to hell, but to tell you the truth, I don't care about it all that much." She still has sex with her husband, but it's always at his instigation, and she said that her libido is "way down." This does not appear to bother her very much, perhaps because she is so happy to be free of the pain of endometriosis.

Types of Hysterectomy

If your uterus is removed via an incision in your belly, you are having an *abdominal hysterectomy*. This is done when either your ovaries or other organs are removed at the same time, or if you have large fibroid tumors or pelvic inflammatory disease. If the surgeon wants to examine other parts of your abdominal contents, or if you have a lot of fatty tissue in your abdomen, your uterus will have to be removed via a vertical or transverse (horizontal) abdominal incision. The latter type of incision is usually done very low (just above your pubic hairline) so the scar is hardly visible after it heals. You can still wear a bikini. By the way, talk to your surgeon before the operation about the incision and state your preferences.

A *vaginal hysterectomy* is removal of the uterus through the vagina, and is done under these circumstances: (1) the uterus is small enough to fit (no large fibroids); (2) there is existing prolapse (dropping or falling through) of the uterus, bowel, or bladder that will be repaired during the same surgical procedure; (3) and the ovaries are to be left intact.

A vaginal hysterectomy may sound more desirable because there's no belly incision, but it's a more complicated procedure and requires a great deal of surgical skill. Also, you will have a small abdominal incision because a vaginal hysterectomy is almost always accompanied by a laparoscopy to enable the surgeon to see what's going on inside your abdomen. A vaginal hysterectomy also carries a greater risk of postoperative bleeding and infection, and there is risk of damage to other organs and structures which might necessitate further surgery.

Preparation for Surgery

Most physicians will require you to stop taking all hormonal medications a month before your operation, and if you still smoke, you will be advised to stop for a month prior to surgery (and if you can last that long without a cigarette, you can quit altogether).

Since your insurance company won't allow you to be admitted to the hospital the night before your operation, you'll have to spend a few hours there the week before having your preoperative tests: blood work, urinalysis, electrocardiogram, and chest X ray.

On the day of the operation, you'll be told to check into the hospital a few hours before your operation is to begin (most surgeons are morning people so you'll probably have to show up by 5:00 or 6:00 A.M.). You'll get undressed, and if no one accompanies you to the hospital, your clothes will be put into a bag with your name, and when your room is assigned, they'll be delivered there. By the way, leave *all* your jewelry and valuables at home. Someone can bring your watch, eyeglasses, and a few dollars for the newspaper the next day. You won't need any of that stuff while you're on the operating table.

When you have donned that darling little hospital gown, you'll lie on a stretcher and the nurse will start an intravenous (IV) infusion, take your blood pressure, and probably ask many of the same questions you've answered a dozen times already. Shortly you'll be wheeled off to the operating suite. Your surgeon will stop by to say hello while you're lying in the surgical suite anteroom, and this is the time to speak up if you have last-minute questions, or if you have changed your mind about the surgery.

This is also the time when your anesthesiologist will speak with you if you haven't already met this specialist. You'll be asked about your past experiences with anesthesia and about your drug allergies. *Always* insist on a board certified anesthesiologist (a physician). Do not allow a nurse anesthetist (not a physician) to give you anesthesia unless that person is attended by an anesthesiologist in the operating room (OR) *the entire time* you are under anesthesia.

Not too many minutes after the surgeon has said good-bye and gone off to scrub, you'll be wheeled into the actual OR and be told to scoot over from the stretcher to the operating table. If you have never been in an OR before, take some time to look around and ask questions if you want. In the first place it's very interesting (although not as dramatic as it appears on television). An added bonus of looking at the instruments and machines is that it will take your mind off your nervousness. And you *will* be nervous. It doesn't matter how blasé you are or how many times you have had surgery, being cut open and having someone poke around among your innards is a nerve-wracking experience. If you don't feel like looking around or talking with the nurses, try lying quietly and breathing deeply to relax.

Shortly after you have moved over to the operating table and are strapped in, you will receive a dose of very fast-acting analgesic (this is not the anesthesia; that's given to you after you're asleep). The needle is pushed into your IV tube rather than into your skin so you may not know it's going to happen, and that's the last you will be aware of until you wake up in the recovery room. If you don't want to be caught unawares, ask the anesthesiologist to let you know before you get the jolt of analgesia because once it's in your bloodstream, you won't know what hit you.

After the Operation

We might as well say this straight out and not mince words. When you wake up from the anesthesia, you will be in pain—bad pain. Surgery hurts like hell. After all, you've just been subjected to a big knife wound. The only "good" thing about it is that it doesn't last long (by the end of the second or third day, you probably won't need narcotics), and the pain medication you will receive really works.

There's a wonderful new wrinkle in the postop pain medication armamentarium: patient-controlled analgesia (PCA). The surgeon hooks this up to your IV right in the OR, and it consists of premeasured doses of morphine that you give yourself by pushing a little button, also attached to the IV tubing. The advantages are that you take it when you need it (push the button before the pain reaches white-hot intensity so the morphine takes less time to act on the pain and is more effective); you don't have to ask the nurse who may forget about you because she's so busy; and you usually end up needing smaller doses less frequently because you're getting the morphine intravenously rather than intramuscularly (a shot in the butt). And don't worry: you can't overdose. The system is automatically programmed to shut itself off when the pre-set dose has gone into your vein.

There's no doubt that you'll feel fairly rotten for the rest of the day of surgery. You'll be allowed to drink clear fluids, and the nurses will make you get up to go to the bathroom, which will hurt like blazes, but do it anyway because the sooner you're on your feet and shuffling around, the faster you will heal and the better you will feel. And it's about a thousand times better than using a bedpan.

The next morning, you'll be hungry (you haven't eaten since midnight the night before the operation), your IV will probably come out, and you'll want to comb your hair and put on a dab of lipstick and a splash of cologne. By the following day, you'll be walking in the hospital corridors (it hurts, but stand up as straight as you can), eating real food, reading your novel, and nagging your surgeon about taking a shower and going home. But stay in the hospital as long as your insurance company will let you because when you get home, you won't have the advantages of a hospital bed with its siderails to help you get in and out of bed, and you probably won't have people to wait on you. Besides, while you are in the hospital, you won't have to look at the mess your husband and children have made in the kitchen.

You could have some complications, either immediately after surgery, a day or so later, or when you get home. The most common is a wound infection, which is serious but easily taken care of with IV antibiotics. Rarely, you could have bleeding from the incision or internal bleeding, which is also serious and might necessitate another trip to the OR. Postop pneumonia or a blood clot in a vein are hardly ever seen anymore because patients get out of bed and move around very soon after surgery. But they do occur once in a blue moon, and both need to be treated in the hospital.

Helen had an incisional infection, which unfortunately had to be opened and drained. This is not as uncommon as hospitals would like it to be (it is *always* a hospital-contracted infection and even has its own medical term: nosocomial infection), and it always resolves itself with antibiotics and time. However, if the wound has to be opened (the stitches or staples removed), it is not surgically closed again. Rather, it is allowed to heal by itself from the inside out. This is called healing by granulation. The procedure is icky (because the wound is raw and red and open and you can see into it), but it doesn't hurt because the skin and muscle nerves were severed during surgery and take several months to regenerate—long after the incision has healed.

Once you're up and about, your bowel function will return to normal, but the first bowel movement can be pretty uncomfortable because your abdominal muscles will not be up to the task. If you have had a vaginal hysterectomy, it will be downright painful. Ask your doctor to prescribe a stool softener (like Colace), or bring your own to the hospital and take one a day beginning the day of surgery.

After vaginal hysterectomy, you may have some trouble emptying your bladder, so the surgeon will probably insert a catheter right in the OR. It'll stay in place for a day or two. Celia said, "It didn't hurt, but it felt creepy—like I had to pee all the time. The worst part was the bag of urine hanging from the side of the bed."

There are a few other complications you need to be aware of, some more common than others, and some more serious than others:

- kidney or bladder infection

- narrowing (stenosis) of the vagina

- hemorrhage, sometimes requiring transfusion

- blood clots

- premature menopause, even if ovaries are left intact

- death, brain damage, or paralysis from anesthesia

After You've Healed

In about six weeks, you should be as good as new. You'll be back at work, back to your full exercise program, back to lovemaking whenever you want, and, we hope, feeling a lot better than before the hysterectomy.

Most women say that hysterectomy has either no effect on their sex lives or that sex is better than ever. For women with endometriosis, if the pain is gone, then of course sex will be fun again. And you can throw away all your birth control paraphernalia. Celia, who is not married and does not expect to be, had her hysterectomy about fifteen years ago. She said, "I had stopped taking birth control pills when I turned thirty-seven, and I was pretty sure that I was infertile, but I didn't want to take a chance so I used a diaphragm or made the guy wear a condom. After my operation, I didn't have to worry about pregnancy anymore so I got rid of all the creams and jellies and made a little ceremony about cutting up my diaphragm. I gave my supply of condoms to a friend. It felt *great* to have 'naked' sex. Then along came AIDS—and I was back to talking guys into wearing a condom. What a bummer!"

There are, however, some negative things about sex after hysterectomy:

- You no longer have a cervix, and some men notice its absence because their penis has nothing to bump up against. Most get used to this quickly, but it *is* something that takes getting used to.

- If you had a vaginal hysterectomy, the size and shape of your vagina may have changed, and this takes getting used to also—for both you and your partner.

- The uterus plays a role in sexual activity. It contracts and moves around during foreplay and intercourse. You may miss this.

- If you have surgical adhesions, they may make intercourse painful.

- If your ovaries were removed, you will notice the loss of estrogen. Consider taking HRT (see the discussion earlier in this chapter).

- If you valued sexual intercourse mainly for its reproductive function rather than just for fun, you may find that the loss of your uterus affects your ability to enjoy sex.

One rare complication that's possible weeks after surgery is an incisional hernia. A hernia is a weak spot in the abdominal musculature through which the intestines may protrude. If they do, further surgery is necessary. If they don't, it's nothing much to worry about. This happened to Helen, who said she had four hernias. Actually, she most likely had one hernia that manifested itself in three or four places. She had no intestinal complications and no pain, but she chose to have the hernia surgically repaired anyway. Her belly looked a little lopsided, she said.

Making Treatment Decisions

Making a decision about appropriate treatment is highly complex and should be completely individual. Because endometriosis is so variable, from woman to woman and in the same woman from time to time, this can be difficult. There are a number of factors to take into consideration.

You should assess the severity of pain and the degree to which it interferes with your life, including sexual function. Your age and desire to have children also will have a strong influence on the treatment you choose.

The extent and location of the endometrial lesions will lead your physician to suggest one or another treatment, but the ultimate decision is yours—and yours alone. How do you decide? The major issue—really the only issue—is the quality of your life, and secondarily, that of your immediate family. Drastic treatment is probably called for if:

- You are in such agonizing pain that your entire life seems to revolve around your endometriosis.

- You are in danger of losing your job and/or your husband.

- You are miserable all the time and you don't think about much other than your endometriosis.

- The endometriosis threatens vital organs or causes part of your body to stop functioning.

As with any disease, the goal is to treat it with the intention of curing it. Because this is not always possible with endometriosis (as it is not with other diseases: some types of cancer, neuromuscular diseases like multiple sclerosis, and chronic diseases like diabetes), the goal becomes to treat it so that it is as contained as much as possible and so that it has the smallest negative effect on your life.

Also, as with any ailment, the best and safest course of action is the least amount of treatment necessary to cure the disease or ameliorate the symptoms. Therefore, if you have mild to moderate endometriosis and can relieve the pain with reasonable amounts of analgesics, your best bet is probably to do nothing. If you are trying to become pregnant and doing nothing isn't working to overcome your infertility, then you'll have to rethink your options. But if you have all the children you want (or don't want any), it's best to take minimal therapeutic action as long as you don't feel incapacitated by the disease.

So the answer in deciding what course of treatment to choose is to decide what you want, what is important in your life, and what your goals are. Then choose what seems to be most productive of those ends.

5

Coping Strategies

Although endometriosis won't be with you for the rest of your life, it's going to be for a long time. Even if you are treated successfully, there is a strong possibility that it will recur (and even if it doesn't, you'll worry about it). That's the discouraging news. The good news is that there are many ways you can learn to cope with the disease without falling into a "woe-is-me" way of life, and without making endometriosis the center of your life.

Coping with Pain

In addition to taking whatever drugs your doctor prescribes for pain (see chapter 3), you need to learn alternative ways to cope with and manage pain. The first thing to think about is your pain threshold. Get to know what it is, and take something for the pain when you have reached it. Pain threshold is generally defined as the point at which a stimulus becomes painful. Some people say that it's when pain becomes severe enough for you to want to do something about it.

It's pointless to be unnecessarily "brave" by trying to fight the pain. You'll end up feeling worse because ignoring or fighting pain is more stressful than taking care of it, and stress increases pain. Besides, nobody likes a martyr.

Relaxation techniques and exercises are very effective at reducing stress, which in turn decreases pain. Meditation can provide a short mental vacation during the middle of or at the end of a busy stressed-out day. It works by helping you block out the outside world so you can go deep into your inner self. Two types of Eastern meditation well known in the West are transcendental meditation and Zen meditation. The former constricts your attention when you repeat a word or a sound (mantra) over and over as you sit with your eyes gently closed. In Zen meditation, you sit with your eyes open and concentrate on breathing. The techniques are described in detail in chapter 6.

Biofeedback can reduce stress and its symptoms by "proving" to yourself that certain mental exercises can lower your blood pressure, change your body temperature, calm your pulse and ease muscle tension. See chapter 6 for details.

Although we'll talk more about sex and endometriosis in chapter 11, it's important to mention here that you need to be frank with your sex partner about what hurts and what does not. When you are making love, experiment with sexual techniques that don't hurt. And remember that sexual intercourse in the missionary position is not all there is to a great time in bed.

Educate Yourself

Learn all you can about endometriosis so you will know what is treatable and what is not, and what treatment consists of. Moreover, you can't make treatment decisions unless you know what the options are. In addition to contacting the organizations and agencies mentioned in chapter 8 and the Resources section at the end of this book, you need to know whether your health insurance will cover the treatment you need. (See chapter 11 for more about insurance.) Also, contact national organizations, especially the Endometriosis Association, to find out about local chapters. Investigate pain control clinics (see chapter 3) if you find that you are experiencing intractable pain. You might even do this before the pain becomes a major part of your life.

Participate in Your Own Treatment

The minute you suspect that you have endometriosis, go to an experienced OBG, get it diagnosed, and begin treatment. Don't deny that there's something wrong, and don't wait until you're in agony and your disease has progressed. The worse the disease, the more drastic the treatment, the less likely it is to be successful, and the more stress and anxiety you will suffer.

If your present OBG makes light of your symptoms and complaints, find someone else. If you are told that it's "nothing," or that severe pain is just something women have to endure, and your doctor refuses to take an extremely detailed history and attempt to make a diagnosis, find someone who will treat your symptoms seriously. You do *not* have to put up with abusive and neglectful treatment from a member of the medical profession.

When you have found a physician you are satisfied with, become an active participant in your own treatment. If you think of yourself as a passive receptacle for someone else's decisions, you will become one. If you think of yourself as not smart enough or knowledgeable enough to know what is best for you, you are wrong. You *are* smart enough, and this book will make you knowledgeable enough.

This is not to say that you should disregard everything your doctor says; after all, you're paying for expert advice, and no matter how many books you read about endometriosis, your doctor still knows more about it than you do and has treated many women with the same problem.

But you will, we hope, be given choices about treatment. (If not, ask about the various options that are available and practical in your case.) The doctor may recommend one or another course of treatment more strongly than others, and you should listen to the advice because the recommendation was probably made with good reason. But in the end, the decision is yours and yours alone. It's your body. You may make a mistake, but aside from surgery to remove your reproductive organs, nothing is irrevocable. (Think of it in the same light as other life choices you have already made: matriculating at a university that, as it turns out, is wrong for you, in which case you can transfer to another school; marrying the wrong man, in which case you can get a divorce; or choosing the wrong job, in which case you can say, "I quit.")

Some women with endometriosis feel as though they have lost control over so many aspects of their lives that losing it in the doctor's office as well is too much. If this describes you, then become a participant in your own treatment; you'll feel better about yourself, you'll learn more about your disease, and you'll develop a healthier relationship with your doctor. Assertiveness is one of the best techniques you can use to cope with endometriosis.

If an experience with endometriosis can be considered positive, Letitia had one. When she was twenty-seven years old, she developed a fibroid tumor in her uterus. "It grew so large that it started pushing other stuff out of place," she said. "And if I hadn't done something about it, I wouldn't have been able to get pregnant." About a year after it was first diagnosed (unusual in a woman so young; most fibroids begin to grow after age forty), Letitia had a myomectomy: removal of the fibroid. "That's when my doctor found the endometriosis."

She had never had any symptoms of the disease—not even severe menstrual cramps—but her doctor put her on low-dose birth control pills to treat the endometriosis. Had he removed any of the lesions during surgery? "I don't know. It never occurred to me to ask, but I guess he did something because I still had no symptoms."

Two years after she began taking oral contraceptives, she and her husband decided to have a baby. She went off the pills and got pregnant "right away." When the baby was born, she went back on birth control pills "for recreation, not for the endometriosis," and four years later, when she wanted to get pregnant again, she stopped the pills and became pregnant immediately.

Endometriosis as Change

A part of your life has changed drastically. Either your symptoms are getting worse and you strongly suspect you have endometriosis, or you have had your suspicions confirmed, and you do have it. Whichever the case, you will have to get used to the change in your physical status as well as the way you think of yourself.

Change is one of the things that most people find extremely stressful. Even a little thing like a new hair style can affect our self-perception for a few days while we wonder if it looks good. But major change creates major stress. The following list outlines some of the things that create the most stress for most people. But remember that everyone is different, so don't feel as though you "have" to get stressed out when one or more of these things happen. By the same token, you don't have to "grin and bear it" all by yourself. If you're having trouble coping, get some professional help. It's the mature, sensible thing to do.

- A major personal loss. The feeling of loss does not necessarily have to arise from death or divorce. When a close friendship dissolves, or the friend moves away, the pain is as acute.

- Being hurt in an automobile accident or other traumatic injury. The more painful and long-lasting the injury, the greater the change.

- Life-threatening illness such as cancer or heart attack. It is as stressful when this happens to a family member as when it happens to yourself.

- Changing jobs, regardless of whether the change was your choice or that of your former employer. Being fired is not always more awful than quitting.

- Serious financial woes. Problems are compounded when your house mortgage is foreclosed or your car is repossessed.

- Pregnancy and giving birth or adopting a child.

- Infertility and its diagnosis and treatment.

- Trouble with the law. Committing a felony and going to jail is more stressful than committing a misdemeanor and being fined, but both are awful.

- A big promotion at work—or any significant personal achievement. (Change does not have to be negative in order to have an impact.)

- Moving to a new house, especially in a new town or city.

Physical Activity to Take Care of Yourself

One of the best ways to get outside yourself for a while and to reduce stress and improve your overall physical well-being (and burn off some calories in the process) is to haul yourself off the couch and exercise. This doesn't mean that you have to turn yourself into a sweat-drenched exercise freak, and get up at dawn to run five miles every day before breakfast, but it does mean that you ought to think of doing something physical four or five days a week.

It could be one of the best things you do for yourself. No, it won't cure your endometriosis, but it will make you feel a whole lot better emotionally and physically.

Types of Exercise

Aerobic exercise conditions the heart, lungs, and blood vessels because it increases the body's ability to use oxygen and thus tends to minimize the risk of heart attack, stroke, and other cardiovascular diseases. Aerobic exercise is done: continuously (without stopping); rhythmically (muscles contract and relax in a regular pattern); in intervals (varying the pace of activity during the continuous exercise session, like fast and slow walking, or jogging and walking); progressively (increasing in difficulty); and for endurance.

Running and walking are the two best aerobic exercises for most people. If you are over forty, you should stick to walking unless you are an experienced runner. Walking provides all the advantages of aerobic exercise. It is free (except for the price of good shoes and socks), everyone can do it, you don't have to go anywhere except to step outside your door, and you can do it any time of the day or night (depending, of course, on where you walk).

Walking is relaxing, good for lowering your blood pressure, and great for getting the circulation going. Aerobic exercise also has been known to lower blood lipid (fat) levels, help with weight loss, increase muscle tone and strength, increase the feeling of helping yourself, and lower the risk of osteoporosis. All of these are effects that we women need to think about, especially as we grow older.

Other excellent aerobic exercises include: jumping rope; exercise classes done with an experienced instructor; rebounding on a trampoline; riding an Exercycle or a real bicycle; using a skiing or rowing machine; and tai chi, a Chinese system which, in its one hundred and eight moves, involves every part of the body.

Anaerobic exercise is usually very intense and uses energy stored in the muscles. Examples are weight lifting and calisthenics. They are not particularly effective in improving cardiovascular conditioning, but they improve physical strength. The stronger you are, the better you will feel, and the better you will be able to take care of yourself.

Flexibility exercises develop and improve range of motion in joints and muscles. These include bending and stretching, which are recommended as part of warming up and cooling down during aerobic exercise.

Intensity of Activity

Common sense tells you that there are various levels of exercise intensity. Taking a walk around the block is not the same as jogging five miles, and hiking through the woods for two or three miles on a level path is not the same as climbing a mountain. Exercise specialists divide intensity levels as follows:

- moderate activity of short duration—walking a mile or bicycling for less than thirty minutes

- moderate activity of intermediate duration—tennis, swimming, jogging, leisurely bicycling, gardening, golfing, or vacuuming for one hour

- intense activity of long duration—football, hockey, racquetball, strenuous bicycling, shoveling heavy snow, skiing, or hiking for two hours or more

Getting Started

Take a new exercise program in easy stages. One of the most dangerous things in starting an exercise program is to try to transform yourself from a couch potato to an exercise nut overnight.

Most women who tend to be sluggards wouldn't do that anyway, but some people, when they make a decision to do something, jump into it with both feet without having a practical plan. They want to turn over a new leaf, leap onto the healthy living bandwagon, forswear all fattening food, and immediately join a health club. This new lifestyle lasts a very short time—a few weeks or until they come limping home with muscle strains and sprains, fall into an easy chair, and say the hell with it.

Try not to be one of these people. It's dumb, exhausting, and hard on your body and soul. Rather, follow these suggestions for easing into increased physical activity:

- Get a physical examination to make sure that you are well enough to begin a physical fitness program. You don't need to make a special appointment with your internist or family practitioner; just ask your gynecologist to listen to your heart and lungs, and mention that you're going to start exercising. You will be roundly applauded.

- Think of ways you can incorporate increased activity into your lifestyle without calling it exercise. For example, park in a far corner of the supermarket lot (walking to and from and around the store could add up to a whole mile), get off the bus a few stops early and walk to your destination, climb two or three flights of stairs instead of using the elevator, clean your own house instead of hiring a maid to do it, put the TV remote control in a drawer and haul yourself off the couch to change channels, walk to the grocery store, buy less food and shop more often.

- Change the way you've always done certain things in order to increase physical activity. Stop driving everywhere and start using your legs or bicycle, don't sit for more than an hour at a time, or go to other people's offices instead of asking them to come to yours (it'll make them feel more important, especially if you're their boss).

- Make exercise part of your daily routine. If you think of it as something you *just do* every day like brushing your teeth or combing your hair or taking the time to read the daily paper, you won't have to think about it, and you'll be less likely to moan and groan before gearing yourself up to do it.

Choose Your Activity Carefully

Do activities you like, or at least the ones you hate the least, while getting the most benefit from them. The best type of exercise for a woman in her middle years is one that uses large amounts of energy over a relatively long period of time, what was described above as moderate activity of intermediate duration: tennis, swimming, jogging, leisurely bicycling, gardening, golfing, or vacuuming for one hour. (Okay, so you don't like vacuuming, but you have to do it anyway so you might as well count it as exercise, because it is.)

Other excellent activities include dancing, rowing, fencing, handball, racquetball, digging in the garden, and lawn mowing with a hand mower (if you have a huge yard that would take forever with a hand mower, trade in your riding mower for a power machine that you walk behind, and don't let your husband do it all the time). If you like to engage in exercise with other people, try volleyball, ice or field hockey, soccer, lacrosse, or basketball.

Stop-and-go activities such as bowling, golfing with a cart, baseball, and some kinds of calisthenics use only short bursts of energy and are thus less beneficial in the long run, although they are certainly not harmful. This means that if you're going to play softball with your office team, make sure you hit a home run every time you come up to bat so you have to run around all the bases!

It is best to do some physical activity every day, but if you can't, every other day or four or five times a week is fine. What you should not do is stop and start an exercise program; that is, get out there every day for a month or so, and then slack off for a month. Physical activity should be a *consistent* part of your life.

Also, you need to think about *when* you exercise. Naturally, you can't interrupt a business meeting, no matter how bored you are, to say, "Sorry folks, I'm going swimming at the Y now." But you can incorporate an exercise program into your schedule so it provides the most benefit. For example, the optimum time for physical activity is about an hour after meals when you blood sugar is at its highest. This is easy to accomplish on weekends, but during the week, you have to make a conscious effort. Try eating lunch at your desk while you are working and then use your allotted lunch hour to take a walk or go to the gym or swimming pool. You won't be the only one in your office who does this.

More and more women work at home the way Kathleen does, which provides a great deal of flexibility about when they exercise—and no boss to look over their shoulders. She is an accountant and often works on deadline, so self-discipline in her work is important. She gets up, goes to her office, finishes the work she has to do for that day, and "treats" herself to a three-mile walk in her neighborhood.

Tips to Increase Physical Activity

Set realistic goals for yourself. Just as you know that it's unrealistic to believe that you will lose twenty-five pounds the first month you begin a new diet, it is unrealistic to believe that you will run five miles a day every day for the rest of your life.

Consider your age, general physical condition, and weight, and then make a plan and stick to it. Do *not* consider the amount of time you have in which to engage in physical activity because you are going to *make* time for it. You might get away with, "I just haven't had the time," as an excuse to your boss for being late with a project, but you can't get away with it when your own physical health and emotional well-being are the issues.

If you decide that you are going to walk a half hour or two miles, five days a week, choose a route in the neighborhood where you live or work. As an alternative to your usual route, scout out a pleasant hiking trail in a park or forest. Choose a time that's most convenient for you (it doesn't have to be the same time every day), and do it. Just as you won't let yourself be talked into calling in sick at work to spend the day at an outlet mall with a friend (well, maybe once in a great while), don't let yourself be talked out of sticking to your exercise program. ("I'd love to go to a movie, but I have to finish up my work and then take my walk. I could meet you at . . .")

Some people like to exercise with another person or in a group. This is one way to maintain physical fitness because if you have paid for an aerobics class, you're less likely to skip it, and if you make a date to play tennis or handball during lunch or right after work, you won't want to be rude to or disappoint your partner.

If you get bored doing the same kind of exercise every day, don't. There's no reason why you can't vary your physical activity (the jocks call it cross training) by walking twice a week, bicycling with a club every other Saturday, and swimming at your health club Mondays and Thursdays—or any combination of activities in any order that pleases you. Consider your exercise program an obligation to yourself as well as a treat you give yourself. Be good to yourself. As the commercial says, "You're worth it."

Don't forget to reward yourself every now and then for sticking to your exercise program. Get a professional massage, buy a new outfit, eat something gooey and outrageous, soak in a hot tub, again, whatever pleases you. And always wear shoes that are in good condition. Check the heels and soles of the shoes you use for exercise regularly to see that they are not worn down. If they are, have them repaired or buy new ones.

Safety

As has already been mentioned, get a physical examination before embarking on a physical activity program. You may be healthy as a horse, but do it anyway. You have great intentions: you're going to shed all that extra weight and get your body toned up so you'll feel good and look good. Fine, but use some common sense:

- Consider the way you feel. If you are ill or don't feel well, don't exercise that day. You're out to have a good time—not train for the Olympics. There's no point in making yourself sick over an activity that's supposed to keep you healthy.

- Consider the weather. Don't go walking or jogging if there's a solid sheet of ice on the pavement. If it's more than ninety degrees outside, and the humidity makes it feel like one hundred ten, wait until the cool of the evening, or go for a bike ride early in the morning. You also can find a mall or a gym with a track, and walk or run in air conditioning.

- If you suddenly don't feel well, or if you get dizzy or begin to sweat more than is warranted by the activity and weather, stop and go home. This is neither an endurance contest nor an effort to see how miserable you can make yourself.

- Warm up and cool down. If you walk, start out slowly and gradually work up to speed. If you run or jog, do your stretching exercises. Take the last block or two of your walk or run, or the last few minutes of the activity, at a much slower speed.

- Dress appropriately. Wear a sweat suit only when you are warming up or cooling down (and outdoors in cold weather), but take it off when you are exercising. *Never* wear rubberized clothes that are designed to make you sweat more or lose "water weight." You could sweat yourself right into a state of serious dehydration.

- Drink plenty of water when you finish exercising, and on hot days carry a water bottle with you. This is particularly important in summer when you have been sweating profusely, but even if it's cold outside and you don't think you've been sweating, you have. You want to avoid dehydration.

- If you travel to a high altitude location, reduce your exercise level because there is less available oxygen.

- Never drink alcoholic beverages before you exercise.

Use Successful Coping Techniques

Think about how you have coped with previous problems (medical and otherwise), and put your most successful coping techniques into action now.

If, however, you find that your life is so negatively affected by endometriosis that you're blaming yourself for having the disease, you're depressed all the time, you're losing romantic relationships, your friends are ditching you, your marriage is in serious trouble, or you're denying the fact that something is really wrong, get professional psychological counseling. Psychotherapy is not an indication that you're a "weak sister." On the contrary, only the strongest people realize that they can't solve all their problems alone and reach out for help.

Controlling Your Emotions

Before you work yourself up into such a bad state, try addressing your negative emotions as they crop up. You probably know what it means to be "in denial." It's one of the big psychological buzz words of the 1990s, and you probably know a few people whom you and your friends believe are in denial about something in their lives. Now it might be your turn: you leave the doctor's office in a state of shock—"This can't be happening to me. I couldn't possibly have a disease that won't go away with a few pills or a little operation."

This is the beginning of denial, a powerful emotional tool. A little of it is a positive thing because it can stop you from overemphasizing negative feelings, but too much can paralyze you emotionally and prevent you from getting treatment. Women use a wide variety of denial mechanisms to protect themselves from the pain and fear of having endometriosis. Some intellectualize the illness and collect vast amounts of medical information on the subject. Some even carry this technique to an almost pernicious end by believing they can manage the disease themselves with various herbal remedies and potions without trying any of the "standard" traditional medical treatments.

Intellectualization is a way to deny feelings and manage stress, and can be used positively or negatively. Learning everything that a laywoman can possibly understand about endometriosis and its treatment is one way to increase control over a situation in which you feel your control is rapidly slipping away.

Some people turn to religion for strength in the face of what they perceive as an overwhelming disaster. Sometimes too much "responsibility" is placed in the hands of God, and you deny yourself appropriate treatment. Besides, endometriosis is *not* by any means a disaster. It is a serious and uncomfortable disease, and you should certainly pray all you want in the manner you feel best about, but you should also take your medications and have the surgery; in other words, do whatever is in *your* power to help yourself. You know the old saw about God helping those who help themselves.

On the other hand, using denial as a psychological technique can have benefits as well. If you deny feelings of hopelessness and helplessness, you can force yourself back to doing what has to be done to treat the endometriosis. It can lessen your preoccupation with the disease, and it can minimize the fear that accompanies it. Denial is especially useful when it results in positive action.

You also are probably going through a good deal of grief; not the grief associated with death, but rather the loss of something important in your life: perfect health, the ability to conceive a child, the feeling that you are invincible. You may be thinking, "Nothing will ever be the same again." You may be right—to a limited extent. Your reproductive system may never be the same again, but that is not the entirety of your total being. You are not *only* your uterus. Therefore, it is appropriate to grieve for the loss of your total reproductive health for a limited amount of time, but it is not appropriate to immerse yourself in permanent feelings of loss.

It is entirely normal and natural to feel angry about having endometriosis. It *is* unfair that you should have this disease. Your anger may leak out everywhere: at yourself, at your mother for passing on the responsible genes, at your doctor for telling you about it in the first place and not being able to cure it instantly, and at the world in general for doing this to you.

Naturally, you're not angry all the time, but because anger affects all relationships, you need to develop strategies for channeling the anger in useful ways. Try to prevent opening old wounds with your husband and other people close to you. Allowing anger at the endometriosis to spill over into other parts of your life will be ultimately harmful. Think of strategies to release your anger in appropriate ways:

- Play hard games of high-energy sports.

- Write down your feelings.

- Go somewhere where no one can hear you, and scream, shout, curse, and otherwise carry on in what most people would consider an unseemly fashion.

When anger and grief are directed inward, they can turn into energy-sapping depression. Not only is this not helpful, it can be debilitating. You need all the strength you can muster to get on with your treatment, as well as attend to the rest of your life. Marianna described hearing her diagnosis as a sense of powerlessness, of being out of control. "Everything else just falls away," she said. "There is nothing in your life but the endometriosis and you think you might never get rid of it."

This is an extreme reaction, but it is one of the ways that people perceive depression, which has a variety of external and internal symptoms: sadness, crying unexpectedly and for no apparent reason, irritability, insomnia (or sleeping too much), decreased appetite (or compulsive eating), restlessness, boredom, diminished sex drive, lack of interest in appearance, and diminished physical energy—sometimes to such an extent that you can't function.

There are ways to combat these feelings:

- Dress in bright, cheerful colors. *Do* get dressed every day, even on the weekends when you don't have to.

- Have plenty of green plants and fresh flowers around. Tend your garden. Living things are reminders of life and health, and they are something for which you must take responsibility.

- Get out of the house at least once a day for a pleasurable activity of even the simplest kind.

- Exercise every day. A long walk with a dog (yours or a neighbor's) is calming, and that tail wagging along beside or ahead of you is cheering.

- Stay in the light as much as possible, especially in winter. Go outdoors a lot on sunny days and keep the indoor environment well lit.

- Open your windows and get fresh air.

- Structure your day so you don't have huge blocks of time with nothing to do. Depression characteristically feeds on itself; keeping your mind occupied with external activities prevents you from dwelling on depressing thoughts. If necessary, write down your activities on an hour-by-hour basis so there's always a goal to be accomplished.

- Plan activities in advance, preferably with other people, so that you are obligated to do them.

- Spend time with children if you like them.

If none of these suggestions works, get yourself into short-term psychotherapy before the depression becomes serious and long term. You might even take antidepressant drugs for a while.

Marianna was so bummed out after she found out that she had endometriosis that she said she didn't feel like herself. "I'm usually a take-charge kind of person, very goal oriented and self-directed. But for a long time after the doctor gave me the news, I felt like I was floating around and couldn't get a grip on things. I was pretty much okay at work, but the rest of my life seemed to be going down the tubes.

"I started picking fights with people, and my lover began to lose patience. She said, 'Look, endometriosis is a bummer, but it's not the end of world. You didn't plan to have kids anyway and the hormone pills seem to be helping, so shape up and stop feeling so sorry for yourself.'

"That kind of did it," said Marianna. "It took a few weeks, but I *did* shape up. Endometriosis really isn't all that big a deal, at least for me, and I hated hearing myself whine and complain all the time. It wasn't the way I wanted to see myself. So I stopped."

Pet "Therapy"

Pets are the most relaxing "people" you will ever have in your life. Dogs and cats provide unconditional love, they are always delighted to see you, and they don't care what you look like or whether or not your hair is combed and your makeup fresh. They love lots of petting, stroking, and hugging, which is a known stress reducer (studies have shown that people who talk to and stroke their pets can lower their blood pressure).

People are often more likely to tell things to their pets than to the most intimate humans in their lives, and pets, especially dogs, are always willing to listen. Cats sometimes need to be in another room, but they'll come around later to listen to what you have to say.

No matter how rotten a day you've had at work, the sight of a wagging tail and lolling tongue at the front door is bound to cheer you up. And the obligation to take your dog for a walk also is good for you. First, of course, it's great exercise, and second, watching your dog sniff along, checking out who has been around his favorite bushes is fun. They are so serious and intent as they go about their silly business that you can't help but smile. And the furry presence beside you or the tail wagging at the end of the leash ahead of you is extremely calming.

Cats probably invented the whole concept of relaxation; no creature on earth has perfected indolence as well as a well cared-for house pussy. Just watching them lie stretched out in a patch of sunshine or curled up in a ball on your comforter makes you feel as though you'd like to do the same. Their soft luxurious fur calls out for gentle strokes, and when they are in the mood for a game, they're impossible to refuse. There is no way you can think about anything else but the cat's antics when they're leaping at you and pretending to attack.

If you are allergic to dog and cat dander, there are plenty of other choices. Gerbils, hamsters, and guinea pigs are a tremendous amount of fun and can be very affectionate. Rabbits are darling pets, very soft and huggable, and they can be litter box trained just like a cat.

Staring at a tankful of brightly colored tropical fish (and listening to the musical bubbling sounds of the water aerator) is incredibly soothing. An increasing number of psychologists, psychiatrists, and other therapists have an aquarium in their waiting rooms.

For people who live alone, a pet is practically essential. For old people or those who are recently widowed, a pet can mean the difference between misery and the ability to tolerate loneliness. It is the fact of their presence in your life, and the need to take responsibility for them that makes the difference.

Helen tells this story about Barney, her huge German shepherd: "Several years ago, he was in the hospital for five days. I thought he would die, but when the vet called to say I could pick him up, I burst into tears of joy. When I showed up at the animal hospital, the receptionist called out on the intercom, 'Barney Reed, going home,' and I cried again. It was the use of my last name as his, corroborating what I had always known: that he is family. When I heard his happy bark as the nurse led him, moaning and woofing in anticipation, to the waiting room, it made my day."

Join a Support Group

At some point after you have been diagnosed, you may want to participate in a support group. Knowing something about your disease before you join will be helpful and make you feel less an outsider, but it's not absolutely necessary. When you join the Endometriosis Association, you will receive names and phone numbers of groups in your area (unfortunately, the association will not provide this information without a membership fee). Also, many women's clinics have various support and educational groups, and you can look in the health section of your newspaper.

Think about the type of support group you choose, and know that if you don't like it or don't feel comfortable, you don't have to stay. There are all kinds of groups. Some are composed of people who just like to sit around and complain, and this may feel good for a few weeks, but in the long run it won't have a positive effect.

Some are so serious and information oriented that you feel like you're back in school. Some provide no real information about endometriosis but are socially a lot of fun. Some are led by people who know a good deal about the disease. Some are run under the auspices of a hospital or clinic, and some are just a group of women who happened to find one another. Some emphasize the psychological problems of endometriosis and some the physical.

There are a number of advantages to participation. Getting together on a regular basis with other women who have endometriosis is both comforting and informative. You may not want to do this forever, but when you are first diagnosed, it can be helpful. Attending a support group tends to make people feel more in control of the problem at hand because they have voluntarily done something (perhaps as a first step) to help themselves.

Reading books and other materials on your own is fine, but if you have questions, and you surely will, the resources of a group gets them answered right away—by people who have "been there, done that." You also derive benefit from questions that other people ask, because there are tips and items of practical advice that you will never get from a book. Moreover, you can take advantage of others' mistakes and experiences. For instance, you can learn how to deal with health insurance companies if you have had trouble with yours. And you can use other women as role models for how to live successfully and happily with even a bad case of endometriosis. Finally, experts are sometimes invited to speak. They are there for you to pick their brains.

Lorraine was in two groups. The first was a support group for infertile couples, which, she said, was a "disaster." There were five couples; four were trying to get pregnant and the woman of the fifth couple had had a hysterectomy. "She cried all the time, and the rest of us were afraid to say anything about wanting to get pregnant because we knew this poor woman never would," said Lorraine. Why was she in the group in the first place? Lorraine shrugged. "Who knows. The group leader was a social worker, but she was an idiot."

She had better luck with the second group, which was women only. "We could talk about anything, and everyone there understood what a basket case you were. No one thought it was strange at all if you said you went to the bathroom a hundred times a day to check to see if you had gotten your period. That was considered perfectly normal behavior for us, and no one thought you were obsessive—even though, of course, we were!"

Avis started her own endometriosis support group. "We had about thirty women for a while, and it was a good group. Some months we had a speaker, usually a doctor or nurse, and some months we just picked a topic and talked about it ourselves."

But she did all the work: organized the speakers, found spaces to meet, maintained the mailing list, sent out all the notices, and paid for the postage herself. "No one would help me. Everyone liked the group, but no one else wanted to do the work, so finally, when I stopped doing everything, it just disbanded." She misses it and would like to get another one going but doesn't have the energy.

Be Good to Yourself

Do whatever you can (and should) to improve your general health so that you feel better. Pay attention to your diet and try to stick to the U.S. Department of Health and Human Services food recommendations: six to eleven servings of breads, cereals, rice, and pasta every day; two to four servings each of vegetables and fruits; two to three servings of milk, yogurt, and cheese; two to three servings of meat, poultry, fish, eggs, dry beans, and nuts; and sparing use of fats, oils, and sweets.

Have your other health problems treated so your endometriosis won't be just one more thing to add to your list of physical complaints.

Don't work all the time. First of all, there won't be any reward in heaven for it—or on earth either. If your boss doesn't like you, working yourself into the ground won't put you in a better light. If you're going to get fired, having been a workaholic won't prevent it. If you leave work on time, the piled-up stuff on your desk will be waiting for you in the morning (and if tomorrow doesn't come, who cares about work?), and very little of life's work is a true emergency. Furthermore, the adage about all work and no play making Jack a dull boy really *is* true.

Set short- and long-term goals in life that are realistic and achievable. Forcing yourself to do things that are impossible, pointless, or unnecessary is extremely stressful.

6

The Stress of Endometriosis

Having a serious chronic illness is stressful. There's no way to deny the stress, but there are ways to cope with and minimize it. First, though, let's look at some of the reasons why women are so upset when they find out they have endometriosis, and then let's examine some of the factors that affect the amount of stress they experience:

- Most women know little or nothing about endometriosis and therefore suffer from serious free-floating anxiety, a general state of fear which is usually worse than being afraid of something specific.

- Many of the things that women "know" about endometriosis are wrong, and therefore they have to correct myths and unlearn misconceptions. For example, one of the most common wrong ideas about endometriosis is that you will *never* get pregnant. This is not a good thing to believe if you haven't yet started a family and have been looking forward to having children. Luckily, it's not true.

- A woman's familiarity with health concepts in general, and the way her own body works in particular, seems to affect the amount of stress she has with a serious illness.

The more you know about human anatomy and physiology (body structures and the way they function), the easier it is to learn about endometriosis, the better you understand the disease, and the easier you can cope with it. So if you're one of those people who needs more information, go back and read chapter 1.

- The amount of confidence people have in their ability to solve problems and make life changes affects stress level. If you can say to yourself, "This is pretty serious stuff, but I've dealt with things that are just as bad, so I can deal with this too," you are on your way to significantly lowering your stress level. But if you are flummoxed by every obstacle that life tosses in your path, you may suffer significant stress when you find out you have endometriosis.

- Age makes a difference. The older you are, usually the easier it is to cope with endometriosis.

- Fear of what others will think when they find out that you have endometriosis causes stress. However, except for your physician, close family (whom you probably want to tell anyway), and maybe a few dear friends, no one has to know what's wrong with you. The disease doesn't show on the outside, and you are under no obligation to explain anything to anyone. Later, when you get used to the idea of having endometriosis and are less stressed about what it means to you and your life, you may want to tell certain people, but you don't *have* to.

- Anxiety over what the disease will cost—immediately and over a lifetime, especially if you need infertility treatment—can get your adrenaline pumping. We will discuss money matters in chapter 11, but for now, suffice it to say that, with the exception of infertility treatment, almost all the care you will need is covered by health insurance. The medications can get expensive if you don't have a prescription plan, but they are tax-deductible.

Assess the Stresses in Your Life

Some people hardly know they're under stress. They bite their fingernails, crack their knuckles, chew gum as if they were in Olympic trials, and can't sleep more than two hours at a time. But when asked how they feel, they chirp, "Fine!" and never realize how stressed out they are. Then there are people who have to lie down for an hour if the cashier was rude to them at the supermarket.

Most of us can take a lot in stride, but on an off day, the least little thing can cause a major "freak out." Be prepared for these times and learn to recognize when you're feeling on edge. We all have different stress tolerance levels; this is normal. Your job is to learn to recognize the things that always get to you, as well as how you feel when even ordinary bumps in the day are hard to cope with.

Most of us live with a great deal of intermittent anxiety and pressure. That is, we don't feel stressed all the time, but when we do, it's pretty awful. This is life—in the big city, the suburbs, and the country—in almost twenty-first century America. Often there's nothing we can do about external factors that cause stress, but there is something we can do about how it affects us.

The first step in controlling stress is to assess it: get to know the things that get to you, and figure out how you allow them to upset you. Here's what most women find most stressful about endometriosis.

The idea of the diagnostic process and procedures can really get you going, especially if you know that something might be seriously wrong, but you put off going to the doctor because you don't want to hear the bad news (by the way, men do this even more than women). Even if you know what endometriosis is, that diagnosis may not have occurred to you because you've been too busy worrying about having cancer. That's what everyone worries about when they don't know what's wrong.

When you finally do get yourself into the doctor's office and the word endometriosis is mentioned, not knowing anything about it may be a source of stress (it *is* a long and scary-sounding word), and hearing the suggestion of a laparoscopy may freak you out altogether.

The best "cure" for the stress of diagnosis is to simply grit your teeth and get the diagnostic procedures over with. Have the laparoscopy if that's what's in your best interest, or the ultrasound, or whatever tests you and your doctor decide are reasonable and necessary. They don't take very long, and the best part is that when they're over, they're over. You'll know what's wrong, you can stop worrying about having cancer, and you will have a basis for taking positive action: treating the disease and helping yourself feel better.

Learning the diagnosis means that you will live with uncertainty for many years, and that's a source of stress that's harder to get rid of. It's easy to allow yourself to become obsessed with the disease and worry what the future will bring—whether you will be able to conceive, when and how much pain you will be in, whether your endometriosis will interfere with your weekend or vacation plans, whether you'll feel well enough to have sex when you get horny, and whether sex will ever be fun again.

You'll probably also worry about how your husband will react to the news that you have chronic "women troubles." If he is like most men, he will probably respond to your endometriosis the same way he responds to all of life's problems, especially yours: he'll deal with it maturely and give you his continued love and support, or he'll have a temper tantrum and behave as if you did this just to make *his* life miserable. Most probably, he'll have a variety of reactions in between.

The way you respond to your husband's reaction is even more important than what he says or does. Louise, who is married to a man who her friends think is a total jerk because he often behaves like a four-year-old (although they don't tell her that), came home from the doctor's office and burst into tears. "What's wrong, honey?" said Lester, all sweet concern and huggy-kissy.

"I have endometriosis."

"What the f*** is that?" angry now, taking his arm away because he didn't know the word. She tried to explain it to him, but he wasn't listening. She also tried to say that at least now she knew why she had those crippling cramps every month and didn't feel like having sex a lot of the time because it hurt.

Lester yelled for a while about how much this was going to cost (they have wonderful health insurance), which of course made Louise cry harder. Then he berated her for not taking better care of herself, essentially blaming her for her own disease. Then, little boy that he is, he stomped out of the house, had some drinks at a neighborhood bar, and when he came home, he refused to talk about it.

Now, a year later, he still won't discuss it and leaves the room whenever Louise brings up the subject. He hasn't initiated sex since the day she was diagnosed, and whenever she snuggles up in a sexy way, he flops way over to the edge of the bed or leaves the room if they haven't gone to bed yet. Louise thinks he has found another woman.

This is a long list of stresses to which you can probably add a few of your own. They exist, in greater or lesser degree, for almost all women with endometriosis. Their existence is not the important issue; rather, it is the way you will deal with them that counts. But you can't deal with them if you don't know what they are or if you are unable to face them. Louise is still married to Lester. When asked how she felt about sharing her life with someone who has so little regard for her, she said, "Oh, he's not so bad. He's pretty good about most things."

One final word about assessing stress: Sometimes you can feel it even when you are not consciously aware of being stressed. If you're getting more headaches than usual, if you have a stiff neck or sore muscles for no reason, if you find that you're breathing rapidly and shallowly or grinding or clenching your teeth, or if you're suddenly tired all the time, you're probably under stress. This would be a good time to look at what's going on in your life, determine if it's endometriosis or something else, and take steps to change what you don't like.

Minimizing Stress

You will need help coping with and minimizing stress. The first and most important step is to acquire accurate and helpful information about what endometriosis is, how it affects *you* specifically, and what you can do to control it. These issues are covered in chapters 2, 3, and 4.

Second, you need not feel alone. Of course, you already know that you're not the first person in the world to get endometriosis, and you may know that it is an extremely common disease, but that doesn't make *you* feel less alone. Support groups are one answer to the problem, and eventually you will want to tell close friends and maybe a wider range of family members.

The third source, which closely follows the first two, arises from your own inner strength. Once you know what you are dealing with, when you learn about the "big, bad monster" that has appeared in your life, and you realize that there is a wide variety of treatments available, it will occur to you that this isn't nearly as bad as you thought it would be. On that day, you will breathe a sigh of relief and incorporate the fact of having endometriosis into your life as well as you have incorporated other things that you wish were different—being violently allergic to cats, for example, or suffering from terrible seasickness so you can't go sailing with your friends.

Develop a Positive Attitude

Developing a positive attitude is one of the most important things you can do, and it may be difficult if you live and work in a highly stressful environment. Because so much of American life is stressful, you have to concentrate on making your own private sphere as calm as possible. So think about trying some or all of the following:

- Decide what you have control over and what you do not, and try to pay as little attention as you can to what you cannot control.

- You will not have control over your endometriosis all the time. It is by nature an unpredictable disease, and the best you can do is follow your doctor's prescriptions and take care of yourself. Once you learn this, and internalize it, you can stop feeling guilty and stressed out every time you don't feel well.

- If you socialize with people you don't like or who are not congenial to be with, drop them. You probably have to put up with your share of jerks at work (everyone does), but you don't have to do it on your own time.

- If your marriage is not as happy as you would like it to be, do something about it. Talk honestly about your feelings to your husband, get into marriage counseling, or get out of the marriage if it's not salvageable. Staying in a bad marriage can put the most cheerful person into a perpetual bad mood.

- Try to increase your intuition and self-awareness, and learn to identify what makes you happy and what does not. This requires conscious thought and a good deal of mental and emotional effort.

- Learn to manage your own life. This is not to say that you should not develop close relationships with other people, and it is not to say that you should not allow other people to help you when you need it. But you, and only you, are responsible for the conduct of your life.

- Recognize that there are many choices to be made in every aspect of life. Too many people stay in jobs they hate or remain in unsatisfactory human relationships because they believe they have no choice in the matter. This is not true. *You* are the captain of your own ship.

- Develop your sense of humor and laugh as much as you can. So much of life is absurd; try to see it.

- Become a volunteer and help others. You'll be amazed at how good you'll feel and how thoroughly your own woes fade into the background while you are giving of yourself to others. And do it regularly—not just a once-a-year effort on Thanksgiving or Christmas.

- Don't whine and complain about your endometriosis. No one except your closest family really cares about your suffering (and even they will soon become impatient with you). Try to accept that. Accept too the fact that you have endometriosis, but you will not let it ruin your life.

Use Stress Reduction Techniques

Meditation

Meditation can take many forms. In its purest, it is a Buddhist religious technique to make contact with one's innermost self. But anyone of any religion can use the technique of meditation, and it need not have anything to do with religion if you don't see it that way. Rather, it is a form of mental concentration that frees you from you usual mental processes. Some people say that meditation, if practiced consistently, can change your life.

Most people don't want to take meditative techniques that far; they just want a short mental vacation during the middle of or at the end of a busy stressed-out day. Meditation does that by helping you to block out the outside world and by taking you deep into your inner self.

The two types of Eastern meditation that are best known in the West are transcendental meditation and Zen meditation. The former constricts your attention when you repeat a word or a sound (mantra) over and over as you sit with your eyes closed. In Zen meditation, you sit with your eyes open and concentrate on breathing.

General rules of meditation include doing it in the same quiet place every day when you will not be interrupted, preferably at the same time each day, and sitting in the full lotus or half lotus position. Meditating after eating or before going to bed is not recommended. Practitioners of meditation say you should start with brief periods, five minutes or so, and gradually increase to twenty or thirty minutes. You should not skip days, and if you really think you don't have time to meditate, it is better to do it for only five minutes than not at all.

If you are going to practice transcendental meditation, first choose your mantra, a short (no more than one or two syllables) sound that you hear as harmonious and melodious. Then go to your chosen spot, assume your position (if lotus or half lotus is too uncomfortable, just sit), take a few deep breaths to quiet yourself, close your eyes, and begin repeating your mantra over and over, slowly and silently. If other thoughts come into your mind, don't push them away deliberately. Rather, let them flow through without letting up on your mantra concentration. Soon you will find yourself in a state of "suspended isolation" in which you neither think nor do. This is meditation. When you are finished, stop repeating your mantra, sit with your eyes closed for a few minutes longer, and then open your eyes, stretch as you would when awakening, and go on about your business.

Zen meditation requires that you use the full or half lotus position on the forward part of a straight chair. Your spine should be straight and the small of your back concave. Pull your chin in and put your hands in your lap, thumbs touching, turned up with the left hand inside the right (opposite if you are left handed). With your eyes open but unfocused, look at a spot about three feet in front of you and downward. Move your torso in a wide arc back and forth a few times and stop at your natural center where you feel comfortable. Sit quietly and concentrate your mind on the rhythm of your breathing. As in transcendental meditation, don't pay attention to the other thoughts that come into your mind; rather, concentrate on your breathing. You can count one-two as you inhale and exhale if it helps you concentrate, but soon you won't need to do even that.

Biofeedback

The purpose of biofeedback is to teach you to consciously control normally unconscious body functions such as heart rate, blood pressure, and respiration. In biofeedback, you are connected to electronic sensors that monitor various vital signs and translate them into audio or visual cues or signals (the feedback). While hooked up to the sensors, you use various relaxation and stress-reduction techniques that change vital signs: slowed pulse, lowered blood pressure, lowered skin temperature, decreased perspiration, and the like. Over time, the techniques are used without being hooked up to the monitors.

Biofeedback has been used successfully in treating high blood pressure, irritable bowel syndrome, chronic constipation, migraine headaches, and other types of stress-related illnesses.

It has no effect on endometriosis per se, but since endometriosis can cause a high degree of stress, you might find the technique useful to calm yourself down while you are making decisions about treatment and while you're undergoing treatment. Biofeedback is particularly helpful in combating the physical and emotional stress of surgery.

Hypnotherapy

Hypnotherapy works only if you can allow yourself to be hypnotized. Not everyone is capable of succumbing to a hypnotist's therapy. It has, however, been useful in treating chronic pain, and it has helped people lose weight and stop smoking.

For women with endometriosis, hypnotherapy might be helpful, not only in relieving pain, but perhaps during the process of making treatment decisions. During hypnosis, it is possible to think about things or come to grips with deeply buried feelings. Hypnosis may not be helpful and you may not be able to give yourself over to the hypnotic state, but it can't hurt you. You will not find yourself doing things that will embarrass you later or that are contrary to your moral, ethical, and social values. And it might be very relaxing.

Visualization

Some people call it visualization and some call it guided imagery, but whatever the name, the technique consists of relaxing and forming a mental image or scene that is allowed to expand so that it eventually fills the entire consciousness. It's one way to relax tension and relieve stress, and it can provide a positive image of what you want to be or do. It can help minimize or control pain in two general ways: first by muscle relaxation that accompanies emotional relaxation, and second by the image you conjure—yourself as a pain-free woman.

Jacqueline described her experience with visualization. "It had nothing to do with my endometriosis, but I've been using it ever since I was diagnosed. Sometimes the idea of having a chronic disease just drives me crazy.

"Anyway, three years ago, I was mugged on my way home from work. The guy who stuck a gun in my ribs and stole my purse shoved me down on the sidewalk as he was running away, and I cracked my head on the pavement. I had terrible headaches for weeks afterward, and finally the neurologist told me to have an electroencephalogram.

"I wasn't really nervous about it because I knew it wouldn't hurt, but during one part of the test, they check your brain waves when you're totally relaxed. Other times you have to be alert and look at blinking lights and stuff like that. Anyway, for the relaxation part, the technician told me to imagine a restful scene and to let my whole self go limp.

"So I imagined myself in this huge meadow filled with wild-flowers. I was walking along with the ocean on my left and a cool, green forest on my right. There were these nice puffy clouds in a clear blue sky . . . and the next thing I knew I was three-quarters asleep.

"It was great, and the technician said that she could tell by my brain waves that I was almost asleep."

Yoga

Yoga was very popular in the 1960s and 1970s, and then it faded out in the 1980s and 1990s when everyone was rushing around earning a living and turning themselves into world-class consumers. Things seem to have slowed down a little now, and yoga is steadily rising in popularity again.

Yoga is a Sanskrit word that means unity, and the practice of yoga is designed to bring the mind and body into harmony. It consists of three aspects: asanas, pranayama, and meditation.

Asanas are physical postures that help stretch and limber the body. Pranayama are breathing exercises that increase the flow of oxygen, which causes relaxation. They both serve as preparation for meditation, or a practice of conscious relaxation, described above.

7

Infertility

Depending on which reference source one reads, women with endometriosis have a fertility rate of 50 to 65 percent, whereas the general population of women has a fertility rate of 88 percent. Among women with endometriosis, it is believed that 30 to 50 percent are infertile, although the true incidence of infertility is unknown. For that matter, no one knows the true incidence of infertility in the general population.

The paradox of infertility in endometriosis is that most of the standard medical treatments for the disease are contraceptive. Endometriosis is essentially an estrogen-dependent disease; the drugs used to treat it deplete the body of estrogen and therefore shrink the endometriomata. But pregnancy also is estrogen dependent. So it's unlikely that you will become pregnant while you are receiving treatment, and when you go off the drugs in an effort to have a baby, your endometriosis will probably get worse again.

To add to the irony, drugs that increase the chance of conception also tend to exacerbate endometriosis. They have other serious side effects as well, so if you feel as though you are between a rock and a hard place, you are.

What's more, if endometriosis does indeed cause infertility, then eradication of the disease should render a woman fertile. Unfortunately, it doesn't always work that way. Treatment of mild to moderate disease does not necessarily improve the rate of fertility over doing nothing. *You* may become pregnant after treatment, but according to statistics, the general incidence does not increase. Women who undergo various treatments for endometriosis, and who also are being evaluated for fertility, have variable outcomes in the success of the treatment on fertility. This suggests that endometriosis affects individual women's ability to become pregnant in different ways.

Incidence of Infertility

It may seem as though the incidence of infertility has increased in the past two decades, but statistics do not bear this out. The numbers haven't changed, but the demographics and attitudes have.

First, the age at which infertility is first discovered has increased significantly. In our mothers' day, childbearing was the province of women in their early to mid-twenties. By the time they hit the magic age of thirty, most women had had all the children they wanted. Now, many women, especially those who are educated and have professional jobs (the ones most likely to talk about and do something about infertility), don't even think about starting a family until they are in their early thirties—often not until they are forty. Then, when they can't conceive, sometimes because of endometriosis and sometimes just because it is more difficult for an older women than a younger one to become pregnant, they swing into action and discuss it openly. In fact, many are so voluble about their difficulty in conceiving that it seems as if there are more of them than there actually are.

Second, for educated, enlightened women, infertility is no longer the shame it used to be. It's a disappointment and it's heartbreaking, but most infertile women don't refer to themselves as "barren" or as failures as human beings. Rather, they take action. They get fertility workups and they subject themselves to a variety of high-tech procedures to increase the chance of becoming pregnant. If some of that action seems fairly desperate, at least it's action. Because the shame has disappeared, they feel free to talk about the infertility and what they are doing about it. Again, all the talk makes the problem seem more common than it is.

Third, attitudes and beliefs about what an individual human being deserves or has a right to expect from society has changed markedly in the past two or three decades. People feel they have a "right" to this, that, or the other thing, and if they can't have what they want, many pout, whine, and talk about it. It *is* indeed disappointing to be unable to conceive when other women do so with no difficulty at all. It *is* sad to go to the supermarket or shopping mall and see dozens of women pushing strollers or holding the hands of toddlers while your arms remain empty. But pregnancy is not a *right* in any legal or moral sense of the word, and it is unfortunate rather than unfair when a woman cannot conceive. Disappointment and unhappiness often muddy thinking, so much so that if you take to heart all you read in the popular press about the problem of infertility, you could come to believe that it is one of the most serious and pervasive health problems in the United States. This is simply not true.

Emotional Aspects

For many women, the inability to conceive is more than a physical thing. It is a source of grief and bitterness, and for a few, it causes utter devastation. If you feel completely undone by the fact that you have not yet been able to conceive, or if you believe that your self-worth revolves solely around becoming a mother, you need to think seriously about talking to a professional psychotherapist.

This is what happened to Lorraine. She spent fifteen years and $150,000 trying to become pregnant. None of the medical expenses was covered by health insurance, and most of the time, the effort to become pregnant was the central part of her life. Her husband was even more determined than she was.

"It was incredibly stressful on our marriage. My husband, who is a doctor, sometimes had to cancel patients and run to the clinic to give a sperm sample, and it's not very romantic to have sex when the thermometer tells you to rather than when you feel in the mood."

But she persevered with grim determination, and six years after adopting a daughter, she became pregnant with a purchased (donor) egg and her husband's sperm. Was it worth it? Knowing what she knows now about the rigors of infertility treatment and what it would mean to her life, would she do it over again if she had to? "Definitely," Lorraine replied. "Giving birth was the most wonderful experience of my life."

Most women with endometriosis who are infertile are unhappy rather than emotionally flattened. They yearn for a child of their own body, but they don't feel as though their lives will be useless if they cannot have one. Infertility—for a woman who wishes to become pregnant—is a physical and emotional burden. It is not a tragedy. It will make you unhappy, but it should not desolate you.

Causes and Treatment

Before we talk about the causes and treatment of infertility, let's define it. A woman is said to be infertile if she does not become pregnant, or if she cannot carry a pregnancy to term, after one year of actively trying by having unprotected and frequent sexual intercourse.

Don't confuse *infertility* with *sterility*. The latter is the absolute inability to conceive or, in a man, to impregnate. A woman who has had her tubes tied, or a man who has had a vasectomy, is sterile. A man who produces no sperm, or a woman who produces no ova (eggs), is sterile. A woman with endometriosis is infertile, and the difference is important to remember. Infertility is reversible; sterility is not. If you are sterile now, you will be sterile forever. (Women who have been surgically sterilized can have their fallopian tubes reconnected, but the operation is not always successful, so for all intents and purposes, sterility is a permanent condition.) If you are infertile now, there is hope that you will one day become pregnant.

Causes

Many women with endometriosis fail to ovulate, although no one knows if this is a direct result of the disease or is coincidental. One thought is that if an ovarian follicle that has been stimulated by luteinizing hormone fails to rupture and expel the ovum, the ovum cannot be fertilized. This is called luteinized unruptured follicle syndrome.

Even if the ovum is fertilized, problems can occur. For instance, when the smooth muscle of the uterus and fallopian tubes becomes irritated, the contractile waves diminish, thus making it difficult for the ovum, fertilized or not, to move along its path to the uterus. Also, excessive contractions of the uterus may prevent implantation of the fertilized ovum.

Other barriers to fertility in endometriosis include:

- Irritation and inflammation produced by retrograde menstruation, or by the endometriomata themselves, can cause an immune reaction and formation of an excessive number of macrophages (scavenger cells), which destroy foreign invaders such as sperm.

- Various autoimmune responses (a condition in which one is "allergic" to oneself) arise as a result of misplaced endometrium. Autoantibodies prevent implantation or cause the uterus to reject the zygote (fertilized ovum). Endometriosis is now beginning to be regarded as an autoimmune disease, like lupus erythematosus or rheumatoid arthritis.

- Increased or overactive prostaglandins can decrease sperm motility. Moreover, ectopic (misplaced) endometrium secretes prostaglandins that affect a number of reproductive mechanisms.

- Anatomic distortions and obstruction of the fallopian tubes, as well as anovulation, luteal phase defects, and hormonal abnormalities can inhibit fertility.

- And—if you are avoiding having sexual intercourse because it is painful, you're not likely to become pregnant.

Although there is no proof of it, scientists believe that certain lifestyle factors *may* predispose a woman to infertility resulting from endometriosis: use of intrauterine devices, especially the Dalkon Shield; cigarette smoking; obesity; and possibly cocaine, marijuana, and alcohol use (Buck, Sever, et al, 1987).

Balance Between Treatment and Infertility

Balancing the decision to get treatment for the pain and other symptoms of endometriosis with the desire to become pregnant takes a good deal of skill and emotional insight. You will need to consider a number of factors.

If you have mild to moderate endometriosis and can control the pain with a reasonable amount of analgesia, it's usually best to do nothing if you want to become pregnant fairly soon. Doctors call this "watchful waiting" or "expectant management." Since most of the medications used to treat endometriosis will further jeopardize your chances of becoming pregnant, and surgery might damage your reproductive organs, you're risking your fertility for very little good purpose.

If you are in severe and/or frequent pain, then you need to weigh the quality of your life with the desire to have a child. In other words, how much pain and discomfort are you willing to bear in order to try to become pregnant? Answering this question requires a long, hard, and *painfully honest* look at your life, your values, your marriage, and your self-concept. It probably will be one of the most difficult things you will have to do.

And then there is the most difficult question of all: How badly do you want, or need, a child of your own body? Would you be willing to trade not being able to become pregnant for significant relief of endometriosis. Are you willing to consider adoption?

Lorraine adopted a daughter six years before she became pregnant. She and her husband are both educated professionals, yet they found the adoption process difficult and expensive. "Do you know how difficult it is to find a healthy white infant?" she asked. She and her husband were not willing to consider an interracial adoption or to take an older child. "And we refused to go to Russia, China, or South America to get a baby. People have had awful experiences doing that." So they waited until a baby of their choice came along.

Avis and her first husband did not have such an ultimately positive adoption experience. They couldn't find a white baby, which was their first choice. "The social worker at the adoption agency asked if we would take a black baby, but we didn't want to. Then she wanted us to take a baby with health problems. I don't remember what was wrong with the baby, but at the time, it sounded pretty serious. So we didn't adopt."

Several years passed, and it became increasingly obvious that Avis was not going to get pregnant so she went back to the adoption agency. "By that time, I had it in my mind that I would take any kid that came along," she said. She and her husband (her marriage was falling apart by that time) ended up with an eleven-year-old boy, and the experience was "a disaster." He had behavior problems from the beginning, and he shortly became a juvenile delinquent. He was in and out of trouble with the police, and by the time he was sixteen, Avis, who was now divorced, had him committed to a mental hospital. From the way she described her son's behavior, it was clear that he was a sociopath.

Although adoption is not without its social, economic, and emotional problems, few people have the painfully negative experience that Avis did. If, after you have thought about it carefully, you believe that adoption is a good choice for you, contact one or more adoption agencies and begin the process. Be prepared to spend a great deal of time and money (even legal agency adoptions involve hefty fees), but in the end you may be lucky enough to find a wonderful child to love and nurture.

If you decide to make an all-out effort to become pregnant, you and your physician will have to assess how difficult it will be; that is, what are *your* chances as compared with general statistics? Of course, physicians cannot guarantee that you will get pregnant if you do this or that treatment. But what can happen is that you can improve your odds with certain treatments.

Types of Treatment

Although you and your physician have to discuss this, combination estrogen-progesterone is probably the best way to begin treatment, if you don't want to become pregnant right away. When you stop taking the drugs, your fertility might be enhanced. Danazol is another choice because sometimes (not always) it improves fertility after the course of treatment. But you must not become pregnant while taking this drug.

You also might want to think about taking fertility drugs. But think *long and hard* because these are extremely potent agents. Drugs such as Clomid, Pergonal, Humegon, Metrodin, and others increase fertility by acting directly on the ovary's function of ripening and maturing ova. There is a drawback to this therapy: triplets are common, and quadruplets and quintuplets are not uncommon (more so with Pergonal than with Clomid; nevertheless, all fertility drugs carry a risk of multiple pregnancy). There was even a case of septuplets in late 1997. In pregnancies involving any more than three fetuses, it is rare for all of them to survive, and even if they do, the medical, social, and financial burdens are enormous.

Lorraine took fertility drugs. "You name it and I was on it," she said. "I tried Clomid, Pergonal, and some others, and none of them worked."

Hormonal drugs such as GnRH and human chorionic gonadotropin can increase the chances of maintaining a pregnancy begun naturally. They act on the endometrium and create a more protective environment for implantation and nourishment of the zygote.

After two years of actively trying to become pregnant, Kathleen began what she called a "low-key" effort. First, her husband Kevin's sperm was evaluated. "It was marginally low so he was told not to wear such tight underwear. I bought him seven pairs of boxer shorts with cute designs on them—one for every day of the week. He hated them, but he wore them."

A change of underwear didn't help, so Kathleen had a hysterosalpingogram (a diagnostic test in which dye is injected into the uterus and fallopian tubes and then X-rayed) and found that her fallopian tubes were indeed patent (open). She took her temperature every day, and she and Kevin refrained from having sex for a few days before ovulation in order to build up his sperm count. Nothing happened so she decided to take Clomid. "On the second cycle, I got pregnant."

Whatever infertility problems she had experienced after her ovarian cyst was removed (and whatever had existed before then that she never knew about) are obviously gone because she got pregnant two more times.

Timing

Timing is an important factor. If you're still in your twenties and you want to begin a family, this is the time to make the effort because the older you get, the less likely you are to become pregnant. This is true for all women, but especially so for those with endometriosis. The progressive nature of endometriosis is hotly debated among gynecologists, and the "answer" seems to lie in the underlying causes of the disease. If it is due to retrograde menstruation, the more periods you have, the worse your disease will become. If the disease is caused by an anatomical abnormality, surgery to correct it may or may not be effective—depending on the skill of the surgeon and whether you develop serious adhesions. If you have had the predisposition to endometriosis since you were in your mother's uterus, chances are the longer you wait, the less likely you are to get pregnant.

If you decide to have surgery (the less invasive the procedure, the greater the chance of preserving whatever fertility you have), timing becomes even trickier. Most physicians believe that there is a postoperative "window of opportunity" that lasts about six to nine months. This is when your luck is at its peak. After about nine months of menstrual periods after surgery, if there are still some endometriomata left in your abdomen, the buildup of scar tissue, cysts, and adhesions will once again impair fertility. This is only a theory; there may be other reasons why you have your best chance soon after surgery, but experience has shown that this is your best time.

One extremely frustrating thing about endometriosis and infertility is that the disease appears to increase the chance of natural abortion (miscarriage). So there are women who can become pregnant but cannot carry to term. Surgery and medication may help correct this problem, but so far no scientific data exist.

Are You Really Infertile?

No woman knows if she is capable of becoming pregnant until she becomes pregnant. If this seems like an oxymoron, it is and it isn't. For example, a celibate woman will never get pregnant because she isn't having sex. This does not mean she is infertile. Or a woman whose husband or lover either cannot or does not want to have vaginal intercourse won't get pregnant either, and she is probably not infertile. So unless you have really been trying without success to become pregnant, don't count yourself out.

But if you have been behaving like the proverbial rabbit and still are barren, your doctor will probably suggest that you begin a fertility workup. Many women who have never heard the word endometriosis first find out they have the disease when they seek medical advice for infertility. The sequence of infertility tests is generally the same for all women, regardless of the existence of endometriosis. It is always emotionally taxing, it can be physically exhausting, and it's expensive. So make certain that you're really ready to get pregnant before you begin the tests. Here's the drill:

- Your husband will need to submit a semen sample to determine the quality, quantity, and motility of his sperm.

- Your blood will be tested to determine levels of hormones such as FSH, LH, prolactin, testosterone, and androgen.

- You will be instructed to test your basal body temperature to pinpoint the exact time of ovulation. You'll have to take your temperature each morning before you get out of bed and keep an accurate record. Ovulation also can be determined by your blood progesterone level.

- A postcoital test (no more than twelve hours after intercourse) evaluates the quality of your cervical mucus and the ability of the sperm to survive in it.

- In an endometrial biopsy, several days before your menstrual period, a tiny piece of endometrial tissue is examined under a microscope to determine if you are producing enough progesterone to permit implantation of the fertilized ovum.

- Hysterosalpingography is an X ray of the uterus and fallopian tubes to see whether the tubes are open and if the uterus is correctly positioned anatomically. The test also looks for adhesions on the tubes.

- Laparoscopy, which was discussed in chapter 4.

- Hysteroscopy, which is done at the same time as the laparoscopy, is visualization of the uterine cavity to look for abnormalities.

- Ultrasound examination (sonogram) can determine the size and shape of the uterus.

Linda doesn't know if she is infertile, but because of the severity of her disease, she thinks she probably is. She's twenty-one years old now and a freshman in college. Her mother had been very ill while Linda was in high school, and Linda stayed home a great deal to help take care of her. "I missed so much school that I didn't do very well, so I just dropped out. Then I got a reputation of not caring about school and not being very bright anyway."

She worked for a while as a clerk in a store. She couldn't get more interesting or better paying work because she didn't have a high school diploma. That and a number of other factors made her decide to go back to high school and finish—not night school to take the qualifying GED exams, but back to her old high school to start where she had left off.

That took a lot of guts. "Well, I wanted to prove to everybody that I could do it, that I wasn't stupid." And prove it to herself as well? "Well, yeah, that too." She's older by several years than her college classmates at a small private girls' school. "I feel as though I'm making a fresh start. No one knows me here. They don't know why I worked for what everyone thinks was a few years between high school and college."

Linda looks much younger than her twenty-one years, and in some ways she is much younger. But on the other hand, her illness and that of her mother has matured her way beyond her years.

She has a boyfriend to whom she seems committed. She says he is very supportive and understanding about her endometriosis. Does he know she might be infertile? "He does. He says he doesn't care, that if I can't have children myself, it's okay with him."

But it's not okay with Linda. "I'm dying to have children," she says. "I've always wanted them. I've always had this idea of myself as a mother at home raising little kids."

What will she do if she is indeed infertile? "First thing is that the minute I graduate from college, I'm going to get married [to her current boyfriend] and get pregnant right away—just to prove to myself that I can do it. Then I might wait a while before having more kids."

And if that doesn't work out? "Then I'll adopt. Or I'll do artificial insemination or one of those other high-tech things that help you get pregnant."

Linda also suffers from bipolar disease (what used to be called manic-depression) and takes three different psychotropic drugs. Therefore, it's impossible to predict where she will be and how she will feel three and a half years from now. (It's impossible to predict the future for any twenty-one-year-old, but for Linda, who's had so much suffering in the past and who exists in a physically and emotionally precarious present, it's even more difficult.) One thing is certain: Linda has the courage and perseverance to try as hard as she can to get what she wants and to learn to take care of herself.

Alternative Childbearing

There are a number of alternative ways for ostensibly infertile women to become pregnant and carry a fetus to term. Not all of them work, some work only after several tries, and most of the time, health insurance will not cover the cost because becoming pregnant is not considered medically necessary. And these procedures are very expensive—upwards of $10,000 each.

What's more, because this is a cash-on-the-barrelhead endeavor, many incompetent doctors have gotten into the fertility business. Some are even downright unscrupulous and will take your money and give you nothing in return. They know that a woman who has reached the point of trying one of these alternative procedures is desperate to have a baby, and they have discovered that such women often are not thinking clearly and making appropriate judgments about who they allow to help them become pregnant.

If you are one of these women, very carefully research alternative impregnation before you make any commitments. Go only to a fertility clinic that is associated with a major medical center or research facility. Check out the doctor who runs it with the state medical society and the Better Business Bureau. When you have your initial consultation, ask for references, that is, the names of women who the doctor has previously treated. Physicians cannot give you patients' names directly because of medical confidentiality, so ask to have a few of former patients contact you. If you are refused this method of investigating competence, do not continue with that doctor.

Following are some of the more common alternative impregnation methods:

- Ovarian hyperstimulation combined with intrauterine insemination is a procedure in which the ovaries are stimulated with drugs to produce more than one ovum at a time, and sperm are inserted directly into the uterus.

- Another method is gamete intrafallopian transfer (GIFT) which requires intact fallopian tubes. In this procedure, ova harvested by laparoscopy are loaded into a catheter (a narrow plastic tube) along with sperm collected earlier and inserted into the fimbriated end of a fallopian tube via a laparoscope. Once inside the tube, the ova and sperm mingle just as they would following sexual intercourse. Purchased (donor) ova are sometimes used in this procedure for women who are either anovulatory or who have no ovaries.

- Zygote intrafallopian transfer (ZIFT), also called embryo transfer or in vitro fertilization with embryo transfer (IVF/ET), is a commonly used procedure. It involves harvesting ova, which have been artificially ripened with drugs. The ova are then placed in a dish with previously collected sperm and allowed to incubate for about thirty-six hours until fertilization has taken place. In another laparoscopic procedure, the zygote (fertilized ovum) is inserted into the uterus.

8

Physicians, the Health Care System, and You

When you enter the health care system as a patient (or client, if you prefer), one of the most important ways to be sure that your needs are met is to be an informed consumer. If you think of yourself as a paying customer of the commodity known as health care, rather than as a passive recipient of a service provided by people who know more than you do, you will be a lot better off. This applies especially to women, who are ripped off, treated carelessly, and patronized far more than men.

Using the phrase "entering the health care system" seems a little pompous—like walking down the aisle or embarking on a grand ocean voyage. And you haven't just entered the system; you've been a part of it your entire life. No matter how healthy you are and how few trips to the doctor you've made before you got endometriosis, you are already a cog in the enormous American health care wheel. It knows who *you* are—that's for sure.

The Nature of Health Care and the System That Provides It

Many people have an almost religious faith in the power of medicine and its practitioners to heal and cure whatever ails them. This is wrong—and dangerous. Medicine is powerless against many of the health disasters that befall human beings. Yes, it's true that an antibiotic will cure a bacterial infection in ten days or so, but microbes are still around. They are out there lurking in wait for antibiotics to fail as a result of overuse, or to mutate into different forms that existing antibiotics can't reach. Moreover, new organisms appear every day for which no drug antidote exists.

And yes, it's true that a surgeon's knife can cut out diseased tissue, and people usually walk out of the hospital healthier than when they went in. But there are dozens of diseases in which surgery can play no role, and medicine stands by helplessly.

Then there are the ailments for which we don't need medical care at all. About 75 percent of the health troubles that beset us will go away on their own with absolutely no medical intervention. Americans tend to run to the doctor at the first sign of an ache or pain, and of course, physicians are more than willing to prescribe diagnostic tests, procedures, and treatments that were probably completely unnecessary—and get paid for their efforts.

The health care system and the practice of medicine have pervaded our lives so totally that we have become childlike in the power and reverence we accord doctors and nurses. They don't deserve it, even if they fix what is wrong. They're doing their jobs: nothing more, nothing less.

Before we go on, it would probably be a good idea to define what we mean by the health care system. It's an American entity that's in the newspapers every day, but you may not know exactly what we're talking about. The system is a loosely structured, interconnected web of individuals and institutions that are in the business of providing health and medical care. And make no mistake about it: It *is* a business—right up there in the top two or three in size and importance in the United States. Who participates in the system?

- physicians, nurses, dentists, physical therapists, social workers, and many other individual professionals who provide health and medical care

- hospitals and nursing homes

- outpatient, freestanding health centers

- health insurance companies

- pharmaceutical manufacturers

- federal, state, and local governments (Medicare, Medicaid, Veterans Administration, etc.)

- pharmacies

- manufacturers of durable medical equipment (wheelchairs, instruments, etc.)

- companies that supply hospitals, nursing homes, and other institutions with everything they need to provide their services

- old age homes

- economists and health care policy specialists

Myths and Misconceptions

Much of what is believed about medicine and health care is wrong, and understanding what it can and cannot do is a first step in taking care of yourself and becoming a savvy consumer.

American medical care is not necessarily the best in the world. It may be more high tech, but that's not always a good thing. We are a gizmo-loving society, so the more machines we see in the doctor's office or hospital (and the less we understand how they work and they more expensive they are), the more impressed we are. In addition, we have one of the highest ratios of physicians and hospitals to people. But machines, technology, and a doctor's office on every corner do not create a healthy society, and except in rare instances, they do not create healthy individuals. *We* must do that for ourselves.

Medical care and technology are not what have been responsible for the generally improved health of Americans in the past century. Most infectious diseases that have been "conquered" are held in check by better nutrition, improved sanitation, and the concept of herd immunity (immunizing vast numbers of people so that when an outbreak of an infectious disease occurs, it doesn't get far). But as the AIDS epidemic has shown us, there are plenty of diseases to which we are completely vulnerable. The death rate from cancer (except childhood cancer) has improved only slightly, and that from cardiovascular disease has not improved.

Medicine is not nearly as scientific as most people think it is and would like it to be. It is, rather, an art based on certain scientific principles. The practice of healing still rests on the judgment and clinical skills of the practitioner. And some of them are pretty poor. It is up to us as consumers to learn about the difference between good and bad medical care, so we can make informed choices about what we allow to be done to ourselves in the name of improved health.

Being an Informed Consumer

Becoming an informed consumer of health care requires a good deal of effort, but it pays off in better medical care and greater personal satisfaction. Let's get specific. You have, or think you have, endometriosis, which is often misdiagnosed or not diagnosed at all. There is no one "correct" treatment, and no one knows the cause. This state of affairs could make you feel as though you are stepping into a quagmire when you make the doctor's appointment. But it doesn't need to.

The first thing you ought to do is learn as much as possible about endometriosis: what it is, how it is treated (and the likelihood of success in treatment), and how to live with it as a chronic illness. In other words, the nature of endometriosis in general. There are a number of sources of information:

- books for the lay public
- medical books, which may or may not be difficult to understand depending on your background and familiarity with medical terminology
- articles in women's magazines
- more than two thousand references on the internet, many of which are helpful and accurate
- specialized health computer programs at public libraries
- medical journal articles, which are the best source for the most recent research and information about treatment
- pamphlets in physicians' offices and clinics and available from the American College of Obstetricians and Gynecologists

- self-help and endometriosis support groups

- newspapers, which now carry more health information than ever before

- local women's health information groups and women's clinics

The second thing is to learn as much as you can about your own case of endometriosis: ask questions of your OBG about the extent and severity of the disease, including a request for pictures and diagrams if you think that will help. Ask what the treatment options are, including all the advantages and disadvantages of each, and find out what the consequences are of no treatment at all.

Women As Patients

Women have traditionally been treated poorly by physicians and other health care providers including nurses, who are mostly women. Things have changed for the better in the past decade, especially in areas where the educational and socioeconomic levels are above the national average. But no matter how sophisticated we think we have become, we still need to watch out for less than adequate health care, because we often are:

- not listened to seriously when we describe what's troubling us

- lied to and not told the full story

- treated without consent and not warned of risks and negative consequences of treatment

- experimented on without our knowledge or consent

- given tranquilizers and sedatives or moral advice in place of real medical care

- given drugs that are addictive or habit forming

- subjected to unnecessarily mutilating, excessive, or damaging treatments

- operated on without cause, especially on our reproductive organs

- sexually abused

Rights and Responsibilities

Patients have both rights and responsibilities. You pay a physician or other health care practitioner (nurse, physical therapist, occupational therapist, social worker, etc.) for knowledge, expertise, and a certain amount of personal concern. But you cannot receive these things if you are unwilling to participate in your own health care and do everything possible to increase the likelihood of successful treatment.

You can derive the most benefit from your physician if you take certain steps and behave in certain ways. First, choose your doctor in an intelligent and responsible manner. Picking a name out of the yellow pages may turn out all right, but it's not the best way to start. A much better idea is to ask people whose opinion you value and trust. This is no guarantee of a happy relationship, of course, because what is good for the goose is not necessarily what the gander likes, but it gives you an opportunity to ask some questions and find out a little about the doctor before you phone for the first appointment.

Find out if the physician is board certified in the specialty practiced. The easiest way to do this is ask on the phone before you make the appointment. When you get to the office, read all the diplomas and certificates on the wall. In most states, they are required by law to be displayed, and if you don't know what board certification looks like, ask. (You also can call the American Board of Medical Specialties.) Do not feel that by asking about board certification, you are insulting the doctor or impugning the qualifications. You have a right (an obligation to yourself, really) to know who you are allowing to practice medicine on *your* body, and physicians expect the question.

Ask the physician about past experience with endometriosis.

Second, know your own medical history and that of your family (parents, grandparents, and siblings), and be prepared to answer questions about it. The physician is not being nosey; your history may be relevant to your health problem(s).

Be prepared to discuss the current medical problem in a rational manner. This doesn't mean you can't complain of pain and other symptoms, but you need to relate the history of the disease clearly and concisely. It's a good idea to write a chronology before you see the physician so you don't forget anything.

Tell the doctor the drugs you are taking, the dose, and how often—even if you think the drug(s) has nothing to do with your endometriosis. Write down the information if you think you won't remember. If you have been treated for endometriosis before, tell the doctor what was done and what the result was.

Third, ask questions about everything you don't understand, and reconfirm what you think you do know. Go to the doctor's office prepared with a list of questions if that will help, and write down the answers. Ask for written reports, with interpretation, of all laboratory and diagnostic tests and make sure you understand what they mean.

Talk to the nurses and other office employees; they are sometimes better sources of information than the physician about certain things.

Fourth, read and make certain you understand all consent forms before you sign them. There is no such thing as a "blanket" consent, except in life-or-death emergencies. You must give written permission for each separate invasive procedure.

Fifth, and perhaps most important, if you think of yourself as an adult who is purchasing professional advice, it is more likely that your physician will treat you as one. Know your rights as a patient and quietly but firmly insist on them. You have a right to:

- Control your own body and be the sole decision maker.

- Know what treatments are planned, what they are supposed to accomplish, their history of success, and the alternatives to what is proposed. This right is legally binding. If the physician literally or figuratively pats you on the head and says, "Leave everything to me," leave the practice.

- Be told all the risks, side effects, and untoward consequences of all diagnostic tests, procedures, and drugs. This too is a legal requirement.

- Ask as many questions as you want. If a physician seems impatient or intolerant of your questions, walk out.

- Protest if you have been abused or maltreated in any way. Either leave the practice (with a letter explaining why) or take legal action, up to and including a medical malpractice suit if it is warranted.

- Be told if you are part of a clinical trial for a drug or procedure that is still under investigation.

- Refuse any and all treatment at any time, even after you are on the operating table and the anesthesiologist is poised to put you under.

- Receive care in a life-threatening emergency, regardless of your ability to pay. Unfortunately, once you have been pulled back from the brink of death, you cannot force a doctor or hospital to provide health care if they are not reasonably certain of getting paid. If this seems unfair, it may be, but it's reality.

- See your own medical record.

It may seem as though (here and in chapter 9) you are being urged to leave a medical practice every time something goes wrong, and that you're being advised to spend the rest of your life searching for a perfect doctor. Naturally, you will never find one, and you definitely should not walk out at the drop of a hat. You should do your best to create and maintain an adult, professional relationship with your physician, but by the same token, there are things you absolutely do not (and *should not*) tolerate.

Remember that if you live in or near a large town or city, your doctor is not the only fish in the sea. You have plenty more from whom to choose. If you live in a rural area or a very small town with only one or two OBGs, unfortunately, your choice is severely limited, and you will have to work things out rather than walk out.

Male Versus Female Physicians

Many women feel that if they go to a female physician, especially an OBG, they will receive better and more sensitive care. This may or may not be true, depending on a wide variety of factors.

Although women are no longer a small minority in medical schools (in many schools they now outnumber men), there is still a good deal of sexism and hostility in the study and practice of medicine—as there is in many other arenas. For this reason, some female medical students and physicians feel that they have to try harder and be tougher than their male counterparts. This can have both positive and negative consequences. You want your doctor to be strong enough to go to bat for you and get you what you need, but you do not want her to be so tough that she has lost all her empathy for you as a woman.

Some women OBGs are more sympathetic of women's health problems, but this is not always the case, and the best plan is to choose a physician on the basis of knowledge, skills, and professional demeanor—and leave gender out of it.

Second Opinion

Getting a second opinion is one of the smartest things you can do for yourself if you have endometriosis. Almost everyone is aware of the necessity of getting a second opinion in many cases when surgery is contemplated (unless the need for it is so obvious that one hardly has to go to medical school to see it, for instance in the event of an ectopic pregnancy or a "hot" appendix).

But if you have endometriosis, you should listen to your OBG and take the advice offered seriously. Then do this all over again with another OBG (not a partner of the first one), because treatment for the disease is so nonspecific in many respects, so "trial-and-error," that doctors look at the causes and treatment of endometriosis in a wide variety of ways. If both doctors recommend essentially the same course of treatment, you can have a high degree of confidence that it might work. If they don't, you'll have to make up your mind what you want to do. Your decision should be made on the basis of the information you received from the physicians (ask point blank why this or that treatment has been recommended) and from your own research.

If you are unable to find another OBG for a second opinion, call the American Board of Medical Specialties.

Women and Medications

Hormonal and other drugs are one of the major treatments for endometriosis, and women consume all types of prescription and over-the-counter drugs in far greater numbers than men. Women also are psychologically and physically addicted to prescription drugs in far greater numbers than men. Therefore, it would behoove you to know something about drugs: what they are, how they are developed and manufactured, and how they are approved for sale in the United States.

Types of Drugs

Drugs (also called pharmaceuticals) are derived from three major sources: naturally occurring substances like plants, hormones, and enzymes; chemicals or other synthetic substances; and biologicals, which are other life forms and include cloned substances. By far the most numerous drugs are those that are chemically synthesized.

Pharmaceuticals fall into two classes: prescription (also called "ethical") drugs and those that are sold without a prescription, known as over-the-counter (OTC) drugs. Just to confuse you, sometimes the same drug is sold both ways; for example, this is the case for many NSAIDs. The OTC version is usually half the strength of the prescription version.

Pharmaceuticals also are classified in two other ways: brand name (trade name) or generic. Every new drug manufactured in the United States, whether prescription or OTC, is originally owned and patented by a private company, usually the one that invested in its development. The law allows that company to market the drug exclusively under its own brand name and charge what it wants for the drug.

After seventeen years (in some cases a longer time), the drug goes "off patent," and any licensed pharmaceutical manufacturer can manufacture and sell the drug for as much as it wants, which is almost always significantly less than its price as a brand name. The drug is then sold as a generic. Its ingredients are exactly the same as its brand name counterpart, and the manufacturing process is almost always exactly the same. After the patent has expired, you will find the drug sold both ways: brand name and generic. Most pharmacies ask which you prefer.

Pharmaceutical Manufacture and Control

In the United States, drug development and manufacturing is always done by pharmaceutical companies, that is, in the private sector. Public funds are rarely used to develop pharmaceuticals.

The Food and Drug Administration (FDA), a division of the U.S. Public Health Service, Department of Health and Human Services, does not develop drugs, and it does not test drugs. It does, however, have three extremely important functions:

- ensuring that all drugs manufactured and sold in the United States are safe and effective

- ensuring that foods are safe and honestly labeled

- regulating medical devices (everything from bandages to artificial hearts), cosmetics, veterinary drugs, animal feed, vaccines, and the blood supply

The FDA was established in 1906 with passage of the Food and Drug Act, which prohibited interstate commerce in mis-branded and adulterated food, drinks, and drugs. This was the first federal effort to get rid of "snake oil medicine" and protect consumers from the thousands of purveyors of highly unsafe food and drugs, many of which were toxic. Since that time, the FDA's range of legal and administrative functions has included:

- control of the manufacturing process of drugs, medical devices, and cosmetics, as well as prepared foods

- regulation of the labeling of the above so that it accurately reflects ingredients, uses, and hazards

- establishment of standards for nutrition labeling and health claims for foods

- regulation of biological products for human use

- protection of the public from unnecessary exposure to radiation from electronic products

- receipt of reports of any medical device that causes or con-tributes to the death, serious illness, or injury of a patient

- establishment of quality standards for all mammography facilities in the country, as well as accreditation standards and federal certification

The FDA has many divisions and departments, but the one most pertinent to this discussion is the Center for Drug Evaluation Research. These are the people who decide which drugs are approved for sale in the United States and which are not. The process takes an incredibly long time, costs hundreds of millions of dollars (of private money), and is extremely complex and often frustrating for the pharmaceutical company. For consumers, the complexity of the approval process and the number of safeguards built into it should be very reassuring. Following is a thumbnail sketch of how a drug is discovered, developed, tested, and approved.

First, a compound is isolated in a laboratory or discovered in nature. Then it is subjected to testing to see if it has a pharmacologic effect. This is done in test tubes and with other laboratory apparatus (in vitro), by computer, or in animals (in vivo). During this stage, toxicologists look for potential harmful or fatal effects of the substance, pharmacologists analyze how the agent works in the body, and computer scientists analyze and assess the drug's properties.

If the agent does indeed have an effect, and if it is thought that it will be effective and safe for human use, then clinical trials are begun. Clinical trials involve testing the drug in humans; they consist of three phases:

- Phase I, the main purpose of which is safety and toxicity, involves 20 to 200 people and lasts several months. About 70 percent of all drugs tests make it through this phase.

- Phase II, which looks again at safety but is mainly concerned with efficacy, involves several hundred people and lasts several months to two or three years. About 33 percent of the drugs that made it through Phase I pass successfully through Phase II. In rare instances, some drugs are approved after Phase II trials.

- Phase III, which is concerned with safety, efficacy, and regulation of dosage, involves several hundred to several thousand people and lasts one to four years. Only about 25 percent of successful Phase II drugs make it through Phase III.

When the clinical trials are finished, the pharmaceutical manufacturer formally asks for FDA approval. The FDA has been aware of and involved in the entire process because at each step of the way, the manufacturer must secure FDA approval for the next step.

The manufacturer then presents its findings at a meeting of an FDA drug advisory committee. There are eighteen of these committees composed of private individuals, usually physicians and other scientists who are leaders in their respective fields. They are not federal employees, and their decision of whether or not to recommend approval is not necessarily binding on the FDA. That agency, however, almost always takes the action that the advisory recommends. These committee meetings, by the way, are open to the public and are extremely interesting.

Before the advisory committee is convened, an army of FDA scientists goes over all the data about the drug submitted by the manufacturer. Chemists focus on how the drug is made, and whether the manufacturing, control, and packaging are adequate. Pharmacologists evaluate the effects of the drug on animals and humans. Physicians look at the results of the clinical trials, including beneficial and adverse effects, and whether the proposed labeling (directions to physicians about how to use the drug) accurately reflect its effects. Pharmacokineticists measure the rate and extent to which the drug's active ingredient is made available to the body and how it is metastasized and eliminated. Statisticians determine if the animal studies and clinical trials were well designed, well controlled, and accurate in safety and efficacy. Microbiologists look at the way anti-infective drugs act on viruses, bacteria, and other microbes.

In other words, when the FDA approves a drug for manufacture and sale, you can be certain that it has been examined and tested six ways till Sunday—and then some. And even after approval, the testing isn't over. Post-market surveys are done, and manufacturers are legally bound to report any and all adverse effects to the FDA.

The entire process of bringing a drug to market, from isolation of the compound in the laboratory to full market approval, takes an average of ten to twelve years and costs about $400 million. Here's the timeline for Taxol (paclitaxel), a drug used to treat breast, ovarian, and other cancers:

- 1971—The compound was isolated from the bark and needles of the Pacific yew tree.

- 1977—Preclinical studies began (laboratory tests and animal trials).

- 1983—The manufacturer applied to the FDA to begin clinical trials.

- 1984—Phase I studies began.

- 1986—Phase II studies began.

- 1990—Phase III studies began.

- July, 1992—The manufacturer applied to the FDA for approval.

- December, 1992—Taxol was approved for manufacture and sale.

A word about clinical trials is in order here. Modern drug testing in humans is not the stuff of 1940s and 1950s horror movies when dangerous criminals were coerced into taking "experimental" drugs in exchange for not going to the gas chamber. Of course, they all turned into ghouls and died a ghastly death, writhing and foaming at the mouth. Those movies were fun to watch, but even then, they bore no resemblance to reality.

Today, clinical trials are carefully controlled studies in which the subjects (patients or healthy volunteers) know exactly what is happening every step of the way. They are told all about the drug to be tested, as well as its risks and known side effects. What's more, any subject can withdraw from the trial at any time and for any reason.

There are two basic types of clinical trials: randomized, double blind, or open label. In the former, no one knows who is taking the active drug under investigation and who is taking the placebo (sugar pill). The group of subjects is randomly assigned to one of these two subgroups (the one taking the placebo is called the control group). Neither the investigators nor the subjects have a clue, and the codes under which the drugs are assigned to the two groups of subjects are not broken until the study is finished.

In open label, everyone knows who is taking which agent. Although a double blind, randomized trial is considered more scientifically valid, there is a variety of legitimate reasons for doing an open label study.

If you participate in a clinical trial (and some of the best and, of course newest, treatment is obtained this way), do not consider yourself a "guinea pig." The pharmaceutical actions and toxic effects are very well understood long before the investigational drug is given to humans. On the contrary, you should consider yourself lucky, and if your doctor ever asks if you are willing to participate in a clinical trial (for endometriosis or any other disease), consider it seriously. There are a number of advantages:

- You're the "first kid on the block" to have access to a new and most likely beneficial treatment.

- Your risk of harm or injury is minimal because there are stringent federal laws and regulations in place to protect clinical trials subjects.

- The treatment itself is free (although the ancillary medical care is not).

- You are doing a tremendous service to medical science—and to yourself.

You and the FDA

The sole purpose of the FDA is consumer protection from harm when it comes to food, cosmetics, and drugs. There are, however, two ways the agency might benefit you directly. The first is the Office of Women's Health, which is concerned specifically with the following areas:

- testing FDA-regulated products in pregnant women

- developing contraceptives that also protect against sexually transmitted diseases and AIDS

- determining the safety of silicone and saline breast implants

- improving the quality of mammography standards

- ensuring that women are appropriately represented in clinical trials, which has been a problem in the past

The second is the various ways in which you can get in touch with the FDA yourself, and get information you need. Contact the:

Food and Drug Administration
Consumer Inquiries Staff
Office of Consumer Affairs (HFE-88), Room 16-63
56 Fishers Lane
Rockville, Maryland 20857
(301) 443-3170

Women and the Health Care System

Many aspects of criminal behavior, such as domestic violence, child abuse, public drunkenness, and drug addiction, are being labeled illnesses. Conversely, many aspects of women's lives and health are being labeled medically. For example, pregnancy, a perfectly natural and normal state of affairs, is now monitored every inch of the way by high-tech medical procedures and equipment that even peer into our bellies to see who is in there and how everything is going. And there is almost no choice for a woman, when her labor begins, except to check into a hospital and be attended by highly paid professionals using even more high-tech stuff.

This isn't to say that a late twentieth-century American woman should never see a doctor during pregnancy and should deliver at home, screaming her lungs out while her husband stands around helplessly chain smoking cigarettes—after he has boiled the requisite buckets of water.

But it is to say that the entire endeavor of pregnancy and childbirth has been taken out of the hands of women and placed into those of the health care system. Listen to an obstetrician talk: "I delivered so-and-so this afternoon." *No*, he did not. The woman delivered her own baby. She carried it, she nurtured it, and *she* was the one doing all the pushing and panting and getting sweaty and red in the face with the effort.

Women's sex lives also are up for free discussion in the doctor's office. Marianna, who is a lesbian, was asked about pain during sexual intercourse as part of her gynecologist's medical history. Because she lives in Washington, D.C., a city with the best educated population in the United States, and because she went to a "downtown doctor" and she saw nothing but yuppie career women in the waiting room (Marianna is a yuppie career woman herself with a better education than the doctor), she thought nothing of telling him that she is a lesbian and doesn't have sexual intercourse with a man.

"What a mistake that was," she said, laughing ruefully, although it wasn't a bit funny at the time. "I never discuss my lesbianism at work. I don't make an effort to hide it, and I'm sure that the people I work closely with know, but it's just not the kind of thing I talk about. It isn't appropriate. But it *did* seem appropriate to answer the doctor's question truthfully; besides, being a lesbian has nothing to do with having endometriosis.

"Well! The whole nature of the visit changed. He dropped the subject of my endometriosis and took up with what he termed my 'sexual health.' Can you believe the nerve?"

When Marianna realized what was going on in that doctor's office, she got up and left—and refused to pay for that last visit. She returned the bill with a blistering letter. "My being a lesbian isn't the least bit 'unhealthy,'" said Marianna. "It's not like 90 percent of the rest of the world, but it's me and I'm fine. I have a good life. I love Karen, we have a nice house and the two best dogs in the world. I like my job, I'm good at what I do—and even my parents have finally come around to realize that I'm not going to burn in hell for all eternity because I'm a lesbian. So the hell with Dr. X."

Lesbians aren't the only women who receive medical direction about sexuality. We're told how to behave during sex, how to have the best orgasms, and to make sure we have one every time in order to be completely sexually healthy. When we express dissatisfaction, we're sent to a sex therapist, as if the problem is an illness rather than poor judgment about sex partners.

Women's lives have been medicalized in other ways as well:

- We see psychiatrists in far greater numbers than men, often for "problems" that do not constitute poor mental health.

- We take more prescription drugs, especially psychotropic drugs, than men.

- We talk to our doctors, not our lawyers or the police, when our husbands and boyfriends slap us around.

- When we have children who aren't very bright, we allow the health care system to give them a sickness label, as well as highly potent psychotropic drugs, instead of simply accepting them as they are, working harder with them on schoolwork, and encouraging their other talents.

- We express gratitude to our doctors for simply doing their jobs.

Medicine has always been an institution of general social control, but for women it has been especially controlling. Physicians have power over the rest of us; there's no denying that. They can treat us well or poorly. They can see us as partners in the effort to be healthy, or they can think of us as children to be cared for or ignored.

We cannot change the way medicine is practiced; therefore, we have no control over the practice of medicine and the operation of the larger health care system. The only thing we can change or exercise control over is ourselves. We must insist on being treated competently and respectfully. We must participate fully in our own lives, and health care is a major component of life. In many respects it can mean *life itself*, and no one has a greater stake in the conduct of care than we do.

9

Relationships with Physicians

Despite what has already been said about becoming an equal partner with your physician in making treatment decisions, the doctor-patient relationship is inherently one of inequality. By the way, the words *physician* and *doctor* are not synonymous (there are doctors of all kinds of things, like philosophy and science and podiatry and optometry, but only physicians are medical doctors), but they will be used interchangeably in this book because most people call physicians doctors. Although all decisions are yours to make, for the most part, your doctor still has the upper hand. Following are some of the reasons why the relationship is skewed:

- You are sick and hurting, and the physician is well and kicking.

- The physician has information and skills you need to feel better and you have to buy that information. The physician knows more than you do about what ails you (except how you *feel*).

- You are indeed the paying customer, but if you choose not to pay (even if the services rendered were way below an acceptable standard), you will lose when the physician comes after you for the money.

- In the case of OBGs, they have a unique power to hurt women, and many of them like to.

- You're naked (well, except for that ridiculous little gown); they are fully clothed.

- The position you have to assume for an OBG—on your back, legs spread wide open, feet caught in metal stirrups, buttocks at the edge of the table (called the lithotomy position)—is inherently humiliating. It's also damn uncomfortable.

- The doctor has gone to graduate school. You probably have less education. Even if you have a Ph.D., you haven't gone to medical school.

- Physicians use language you don't understand (medicalese) and won't translate unless you ask—over and over again.

- They use the parent-child relationship as a model for "managing" patients, which automatically puts the patient at a disadvantage. Even the word *manage* is patronizing and condescending.

- They expect trust, even demand it, before they have earned it, and sometimes despite the fact that they are untrustworthy.

- They call you by your first name and expect to be referred to as "Dr. So-and-So."

We Are Partly to Blame

Over the decades in our relationships with physicians, especially OBGs, we women have become adept at blaming ourselves when the relationship is less than satisfactory. We have devised many ways to shoot ourselves in the foot. We feel immature and stupid for being embarrassed or humiliated about exposing ourselves in front of a relative stranger, or a total stranger, the first time. What we are required to do *is* embarrassing and humiliating, and most of us have to force ourselves to do it.

We have unrealistic expectations of our doctors, and then we get angry and hurt when those expectations aren't met. Your doctors aren't your friends, they probably aren't too interested in your nonmedical problems (they are trained to take care of your medical problems, not your emotional and social ones), and will never be able to give you total reassurance that everything will be all right. Moreover, doctors are only doctors, not walking medical encyclopedias, and there's no way they will know everything about endometriosis. The best you can expect from any physician is competent treatment, a pleasant bedside manner, and admission to being stumped when that is the case.

We refuse to complain of pain that we have been subjected to unnecessarily or unexpectedly, and we assume that whatever judgment physicians make must be right because they have better education, training, and knowledge than we do, and that medical decisions are always made in the patient's best interest. The former is an erroneous assumption. Medical school is not high-level education, and physicians are not particularly well-educated people. In order to get through medical school, one needs a terrific short-term memory and the ability to master enormous detail until the exams are over. (By the way, the characteristics that create a good medical student are not the ones that make a good physician.) Your doctor knows more about a very narrow field of endeavor than you do, and that's it. You are *not* in any way inferior to your doctor.

The latter assumption about medical decisions is often, but not always, true. Many patients are subjected to procedures that are either medically questionable or downright unnecessary because they bring in revenue, and health insurance companies don't balk at reimbursing for such procedures if the physician is adept at justifying them.

If we are hustled out of the office before we get all our questions answered, we feel guilty for wasting so much of their valuable time, even though we are paying for that time. The same goes for being kept waiting long past the appointment time. Most physicians schedule a patient every fifteen minutes even though they are well aware that most visits take far longer than that. Some doctors even schedule two patients for the same time slot.

Many offer gratuitous advice about other than medical aspects of our lives, and we don't tell them it's none of their business. And we don't correct them when they call us "hon" or "dear."

And perhaps the worst of our "sins" when it comes to relationships with our OBGs, is that we hold them in awe and are intimidated by them. We're grateful when they treat us well, and we make excuses for them when they treat us badly. We often don't tell the truth about what we've been doing (or not doing) because we don't want them to think badly of us, or we don't want to appear foolish or stupid. We don't ask for a second opinion for fear of giving offense. In this respect, we use a BIG gun to shoot ourselves in the foot.

Creating a Satisfactory Relationship

Instead of feeling wretched and guilty over the way your doctor treats you, instead of having a drink or bursting into tears, or instead of voting with your feet and looking for another physician (unless yours is incompetent and/or cruel), take steps to improve the relationship and put it on a more mature and equal footing.

Tell your doctor what you expect from the relationship. Ideally, this should be done at the first visit, but there's no reason why it can't be done on subsequent visits.

Marianna tells the following story as an example: "Many years ago, I woke up in the middle of the night with an excruciating stabbing pain in my eye. It felt like someone had stuck an ice pick in there. I called my ophthalmologist who told me that he didn't make house calls and to go to the emergency room. I was treated there by a resident who didn't seem to know much about eyes, but luckily it was only a corneal abrasion, and analgesic eye drops and time healed it. The next morning, I called my doctor and told him that I understood about the house calls, but that if he didn't want to deal with emergencies (he should have showed up in the emergency room to treat me), he was in the wrong business. I said that when I needed him, I needed *him*, and that I expected him to be available in a crisis. He apologized, and I stayed with him until I moved out of town."

Discuss charges before a procedure is performed. Ask if the doctor engages in balance billing (the practice of billing the patient for the balance of the bill after insurance reimbursement), and be frank about the fact that you will not pay more than the reasonable and customary charges set by your insurance company. Stick to your guns; don't be intimidated by threats of a collection agency. The easiest way to deal with the issue of balance billing is not to go to a doctor who will not deal with your health insurance carrier.

Ask at which hospitals they have admitting privileges. If a physician is on the admitting staff of only one hospital and you have had a bad experience and don't want to be a patient there again, you may not be able to continue with this doctor if there is a likelihood that you'll end up in the hospital. Unless you are pretty certain that you will need surgery, this is not as big a handicap as it appears. But if an operation looms in your future, tell the doctor why you won't go to that hospital, and you may be referred to a colleague with admitting privileges at another hospital. Of course, if you live in a rural area or a small town with only one hospital, this is a moot point.

Behave like a grown-up woman and you will probably be treated like one. You may feel as though you are being lectured to by your mother right about now, but she would have agreed with the following advice: Even if you feel like wringing your hands in anguish, don't do it in front of the doctor. Talk about your history and symptoms in a measured and rational way. You don't have to *feel* rational, but you'll be taken more seriously if you act sensibly. A calm demeanor also helps you tell your story coherently so the doctor can get an accurate picture of what the problem is.

Ask all the questions you want. It's a good idea to write them down beforehand because no matter how positive the relationship or how professional the physician, just being there will fluster you. Also, write down the answers to your questions and do it in front of the doctor. It'll prevent you from forgetting everything you've been told, and it will make you look serious and interested in yourself. And do not leave the office until *you* are finished with the visit, all your questions have been answered and you understand everything that has happened. If the physician stands up or otherwise signals that the time is up, sit there until you get what you need. This is hard to do, but it's a technique worth learning. You also can use it on your boss and co-workers if you need to. In fact, you can use them to practice on (don't let them know what you're doing, of course), so you won't feel so nervous when you get to the doctor's office. You might even ask your husband or an older child to role-play with you. Explain what you want to do and why, and they'll probably get into the spirit of the game and be happy to help.

Follow the doctor's orders and do what has been prescribed. Take your medicine, do the exercises, don't eat what you're not supposed to eat, get the X ray or blood test. If you don't take care *of* yourself, you send a silent but strong message that you don't care *about* yourself.

Don't ask your own physician to recommend someone for a second opinion, and don't use a partner. Try to see someone on the staff at another hospital.

Marianna, who can be a tough cookie when she needs to be, had to make a decision about her present internist: "Every time I went to the office, my blood pressure went off the charts. Luckily, I go only about once a year because there's nothing wrong with me except my endometriosis, and my gynecologist takes care of that.

"There are two things that drive me absolutely crazy. The first is the office staff. It's hard to imagine a bunch of ruder, stupider, more insensitive people. I know that medical office receptionists are kind of horrible in general, but these women take the cake! The second thing is that the doctor is *always* late. Sometimes I've waited an hour.

"Every time I see the doctor, I complain about the way she runs her office, but she just shrugs (the office workers are probably nice to *her*) and makes excuses for them: this one had a hard life, and that one's husband left her—that kind of nonsense. Once I wrote a letter to the managing partner in the practice, but I got no response. My feeling is that this sort of stuff doesn't justify incompetence and rudeness at work, but I'm beginning to think I'm the only person left in the United States who feels that way. She also said that she's the kind of doctor who takes time with her patients and 'just always runs late.'

"Anyway, it finally dawned on me that things weren't going to change, and I had two choices: accept it or leave. I like the doctor; she takes me seriously, she's smart, she listens, and she always returns calls. She cares about her patients and tries her best. And compared to some of the numbskulls practicing medicine out there, she's great, so I considered myself lucky. I decided to stay.

"Now I make the first or second appointment in the morning and don't wait more than fifteen minutes, and I try not to pay attention to the women who run the place. And the less time I have to sit in the waiting room, the less aggravated I am so my blood pressure is perfect when I finally get to see the doctor!"

Special Considerations in Endometriosis

Choosing an OBG for general gynecologic check-ups, or for obstetrical care, is one thing. Choosing one to treat your endometriosis is quite another. Following are some of the considerations you might think about when picking an OBG—or continuing with the one you already have.

- Endometriosis is going to be with you for a while, and you're going to making more than your usual number of visits to the doctor. You'll be in the office often and developing a closer relationship than you have had before, or that you may have had with other medical specialists.

- It's possible that this physician will operate on you, so you ought to have confidence in the surgical ability and skill in comforting you and taking care of you while you are going through a stressful time.

- The intensity of the experience of having endometriosis may be new to you, and you need to be assured that your doctor understands what you are going through and will provide the emotional support you need.

- Having endometriosis may involve making some life-altering decisions, such as having a hysterectomy, deciding to adopt a child, going through a fertility workup. You need a doctor who can provide the factual information that you will need to make big decisions, as well as the understanding to help you see the various risks and benefits.

- You need to feel as though you can easily communicate your thoughts and feelings about the disease and its treatment.

Linda's experience with her gynecologist has been a mixed bag. When her symptoms began, at the same time her menstrual periods began, her mother took her to a female gynecologist who put the fifteen-year-old girl on oral contraceptives without telling either Linda or her mother that she suspected endometriosis.

Linda took the combination hormone therapy for four years until she had a bad reaction to them, at which time she was switched to a monthly injection of Depo-Provera. Still, she was not diagnosed with endometriosis, and the gynecologist never suggested laparoscopic surgery to confirm what she probably strongly suspected.

For almost six years, Linda had a variety of abdominal and pelvic symptoms: severe pain during menstruation, serious and frequent bladder infections (up to twenty a year, she said), and pernicious diarrhea that left her weak and dehydrated. She was exhausted all the time and often had a low-grade fever. She had a barium enema and a colonoscopy, which revealed nothing wrong with her intestines—at least on the inside.

It was when an emergency room nurse told her that she looked like someone with endometriosis, Linda heard the word and told her gynecologist what the nurse had said. And it wasn't until she had the laparoscopic surgery that she received pain medication that worked.

Linda likes her gynecologist, a woman, trusts her, and feels she can discuss things with the doctor. "All the doctors in the emergency room were male, and they didn't understand what was going on with me, and they didn't want to help me."

Gender probably isn't the significant issue here. Linda has not been treated appropriately. Perhaps the gynecologist, knowing how rare endometriosis is in someone as young as Linda, did not do what should have been done to make the diagnosis early, but that is no excuse for not making a correct diagnosis. If she had, Linda would have been saved from years of pain and suffering—both physical and mental. She would not have suffered at the hands of the emergency room physicians who also did not put the signs and symptoms together in order to find the endometriosis.

On the other hand, now that the diagnosis has been made, surgery performed, and reasonably effective hormonal therapy instituted, Linda has confidence that her gynecologist will care for her well.

You *Make the Choices*

Don't forget that choice is a powerful tool. *You* choose your physician and *you* choose to stay. Most people find a physician through referrals from friends or relatives. If you are new to an area, ask around about a doctor who people seem satisfied with. Ask yourself what's important to you in a physician: male or female, old or young, office location, office hours, personality, type of practice (for example, solo or group, although you won't find the former much anymore.) And by the way, doctors know how they build their business, so if you leave a practice, the doctors there know they won't get another drop of business from you and might even lose business because of what you have complained about.

Stay informed about your endometriosis and the rest of your health care. Request an explanation of the various blood, urine, and other tests your physicians do, and make certain you understand what they mean. Doctors are professionals and most of the time know what they are doing. However, this does not mean that you are less smart than your doctor or that you know less about certain things. For instance, you are the only one who knows how you feel, and you are the one with the endometriosis. Also, you are the one paying the bills. Although you are not technically the employer of your physicians, they are working for you because in a very real sense you are buying their professional services. If you are dissatisfied with the service, or if you don't like a physician, find another one. You are not in any way obligated to stay with them. If you hurt their feelings by leaving the practice (an unlikely event), so what?

Following are some of the common reasons why people tend to leave a medical practice:

- Physicians don't listen or pay attention to what you are saying. They don't make notes in your medical record about what you say and feel.

- Your questions aren't answered to your complete satisfaction, or when your physician answers questions, you don't understand the language.

- You never find out why you need a certain test, procedure, or medication, and your doctor doesn't tell you the dangers and negative effects of procedures and medicines.

- You feel rushed through the visit, and the physician is too busy to give you all the time you need.

- They don't return phone calls.

- A physician has been drinking—even in the middle of the night. Physicians on call are not allowed to drink.

- Your physician refuses to make accommodations about money: reducing the amount of the bill if you are short of funds, or allowing you to pay off the bill a little at a time.

- The physician becomes belligerent or defensive if you say you want a second opinion, or if you object to a certain treatment, or ask what the options are to a recommended treatment. This is an insecure and therefore dangerous practitioner, and you should leave at once.

Laurel saw a number of OBGs before she found one who took her endometriosis seriously. "They all told me, either in so many words, or they implied it, that the pain was all in my head, and that made me furious. I refuse to stay with a doctor who doesn't believe what I'm saying. Did they all think I was faking when they saw me doubled over in pain and retching?"

If you have decided to leave your physician, don't to it until you have found another one. A physician is obligated to treat you as long as you are a patient in the practice (refusal to do so is considered abandonment and is unethical and illegal), but once you leave the practice, that obligation ceases. So don't leave yourself in the lurch. You never know when an emergency will crop up.

If All Else Fails

Before you walk out in a huff, however, think about what went wrong and whether the relationship might be salvaged. Finding another doctor when you are ill and feeling vulnerable is a stressful and difficult task. Do you simply not like the physician, or were you a victim of incompetence or malpractice? The former is a perfectly justifiable reason to leave, but ask yourself if this is the best time to do it. If the latter is the problem, you have recourse, as explained below.

If you believe you have been a victim of medical malpractice (difficult to prove even if you have been seriously and permanently harmed), there are steps you can take:

- First, get a copy of your medical record. You will be charged a small fee for photocopying (when the bill for copying arrives, don't let yourself be soaked; refuse to pay more than you would have fed into a machine at a discount stationery store). Make certain the record is complete; when you go to the office to pick it up, compare what you have been given with the original—page for page. The office staff may give you a hard time about this and tell you that they're not allowed to let you see the original. This is baloney. It's *your* record, and as long as you don't take the original out of the office, there's no reason why you can't look at it.

- Document (with photographs if appropriate) in writing everything that happened. Describe dispassionately and clearly, in chronological order, what led up to the charge of malpractice, the nature of the error or malpractice, and what you have done to remedy whatever the doctor did. If there were witnesses, get their names, addresses, and phone numbers—just as you do in an automobile accident.

- Send all this to the doctor with a copy to the state board of medical licensure and the ethics committee of the local medical society (state, county, or municipal). If the physician is a board certified OBG, send a copy to the American College of Obstetricians and Gynecologists. If the doctor is part of a large group practice, send a copy to the managing partner.

- If you feel as though you have not been satisfied by these organizations, contact a medical malpractice attorney. A reputable one who won't charge you an arm and a leg is difficult to find. Try to get a reference from friends or acquaintances, but *don't* hire one who advertises on late night television or on the back of the phone book. Also, make certain the attorney will take the case on contingency, and don't be surprised if you are discouraged from suing the doctor. But if you have a good case, you may emerge from what has been a very unpleasant and stressful situation with a sizeable chunk of money as the result of an out-of-court settlement.

If you do decide to change physicians, be frank about why. Doctors need to know why patients are dissatisfied, and there may be an effort to right wrongs. Give the doctor the benefit of the doubt unless you have been seriously emotionally or physically mistreated. When you leave, settle your account. If you owe money, the physician may not be willing to send your records to the new doctor.

10

Alternative Medicine

A recent article in the *New England Journal of Medicine* (Eisenberg, 1993) reported that more than a third of the people surveyed said they use "unconventional therapy," which is defined as medical treatments neither taught in U.S. medical schools nor generally practiced by American physicians. A more common term is alternative medicine. In addition, Americans made 425 million visits to alternative medical practitioners and only 388 million visits to primary care physicians in one recent year. The total cost of alternative therapy was $13.7 billion, of which $10.3 billion was not reimbursed by health insurance.

These numbers tell a significant story. Americans are willing to spend time and money on healing techniques that are unscientific, unproven, and which make most physicians throw up their hands in horror. Why?

The reasons are numerous and complex. Mainstream (traditional) medicine is expensive and relies on drugs, surgery, and high technology. However, alternative care may be no cheaper if you have to pay for it entirely out of your own pocket, and many alternative practitioners use or prescribe a variety of pills, most of which have not been approved by the Food and Drug Administration, in addition to using potions, herbs, and mechanical devices. But they are different from what we usually see in the doctor's office, so that may be one of the appeals.

People complain that traditional medicine is fragmented, shuns us from specialist to specialist, and leaves us feeling as if we are traveling on an assembly line. This is surely true, and alternative practitioners tout the advantage of "holistic" healing. However, in modern medicine, it is impossible to know everything about what ails the human body, and often a specialist is called for. For instance, it is highly unlikely that an herbalist or naturopath will be able to do one thing for your endometriosis, although you may come out of the office with a recommendation for a healthier diet and some potions to calm your frazzled nerves.

On the other hand, whatever healing techniques or medical interventions one experiences, the more effective they will be if we cooperate with and encourage the process by our willingness to be healed or cured. Stories abound about people's courage and ability to prevail in the face of devastating illness or disease—even in the face of "certain" death.

People with chronic illnesses, including, and perhaps especially, women with endometriosis, become frustrated by the inability of mainstream medicinal practitioners to cure them. This is not rational, but it is understandable. So they rush to alternative healers in the vain hope of a cure. And women use alternative medicine in far greater numbers than men.

Having said all this, it should not be construed that all alternative medicine is equally bad—or equally acceptable. Some practitioners are well intentioned and will not hurt you. Some might even help. But there are practitioners all over the place peddling weird, quick-fix remedies that will do nothing but shrink your wallet. Because endometriosis is such an "on-again, off-again" type of disease, women who have it tend to become discouraged by the failure of the first or second treatment they try. Therefore, many of them try alternative healing techniques at some point.

If you are thinking about using alternative medicine, the following suggestions might protect you from the worst abuses:

- Look askance at personal endorsements: "Jane lost thirty pounds in a month with such-and-such diet remedy," or "Dick has been pain free for a year after using the so-and-so machine." Jane and Dick might indeed have lost weight or feel better, but it's probably not the result of the advertised claim. Personal anecdotes can never take the place of scientific testing.

- If you feel that an alternative practitioner is trying to hoodwink you or is making ridiculous claims, you're probably right. Leave the office.

- Don't be fooled by fancy titles or degrees on the wall. Someone is either a physician or is not. And a physician is either licensed by the state or is not. Look at the diplomas and license (most states require them to be displayed, and all reputable physicians do it anyway), and if you don't recognize the educational institution or licensing body, ask what the framed certificates mean.

- Make certain you understand all the risks and side effects of the treatment you are about to submit to. All medical treatment, regardless of who provides it, carries risk and you have a right to know what it is. If the practitioner tells you that it is "absolutely safe" or "guaranteed to heal," leave the office. It's a lie.

- If you have to pay for the treatment up front or are required to make a deposit before your appointment, find someone else. Does a restaurant require you to pay for the meal before you eat it?

The Nature of Alternative Healing

Most forms of alternative healing or alternative medicine are lumped together in an approach called "holistic" health care. That is, the goal of the practitioner is to treat the patient as a whole person rather than an ailing body part. This sounds lovely and desirable, and in a purely theoretical sense, it is. But with few exceptions, it is not the way most alternative practitioners practice. Most make a diagnosis, prescribe a treatment, and then send you a bill, just like mainstream medical practitioners. Their scope of practice may be different but the methods are similar.

Endometriosis is a good case in point. A certain body system has gone awry, but the disease affects your entire life—including close personal relationships. It *should* be treated holistically, but there is no reason why kind, caring, and competent gynecologists can't do this. Plus, you have the added benefit of their specialized knowledge of the female reproductive system. It is highly unlikely that you will get both these crucial components of endometriosis care from an alternative healer.

One philosophy of holistic health care is that most of us are healthy in body and mind, and that we exist in a state of being that seeks balance (homeostasis) but is in a constant state of flux. Again, this sounds fine, but if we were so healthy, we wouldn't need to spend our money on doctors—holistic, alternative, or traditional. Again, let's use the example of endometriosis: You have a disease, or at least you think you do, and otherwise you feel great. You don't need to go to the doctor for the "great" part; you need to get the diseased part diagnosed and fixed. Holistic or alternative health care probably can't do this for you, although it may not do you much harm either.

Holistic care emphasizes self-healing based on the fact that our bodies exist in a constant state of breakdown and repair. This is true, but it happens without outside intervention. Our cells die and regenerate (except brain cells) by themselves. For example, a cut forms a scab, which dries up and falls off to reveal new, healthy tissue. Or, we fall into despair over the death of a loved one, and slowly we recover. It is true that these things happen, but they do so without the assistance of the medical establishment—traditional or alternative. Sometimes, alternative healing techniques can boost the body's and mind's own healing powers, but not always.

Many nontraditional healers use the word "energy" when they talk about what they do. They don't mean electric power or rays of sunlight. They seem to refer to some source that human beings have within themselves that can be used for strength, for healing, for power. Whatever this energy is, we all have it, although we call it by many different names such as soul, will, spirit, essence, anima, and breath of life. But it is this aspect of our nature that figures prominently in almost all types of alternative healing.

Treatments That Can Be Beneficial

Acupuncture

Acupuncture is one of the most widely accepted alternative therapies, and some mainstream physicians even recommend it for patients in pain. In late 1997, an advisory committee of the Food and Drug Administration acknowledged that acupuncture does indeed have therapeutic value. This may not sound like a big deal, but it is. The FDA is an extremely cautious agency chartered to ensure that drugs, medical devices, and other treatments are safe and effective. Therefore, you can feel confident that a treatment modality that receives its imprimatur is indeed safe and effective. Moreover, you are now more likely to get your health insurance carrier to reimburse for acupuncture.

Acupuncture, which originated in China more than 2,000 years ago, involves insertion of very fine needles into certain points on the skin, the purpose of which is to unblock and balance the flow of life force through the body. Some traditional physicians, while acknowledging the efficacy of acupuncture, attribute its effectiveness to the release of endorphins, a naturally occurring chemical that acts as an analgesic.

If you visit an acupuncturist for endometriosis, you will find an approach to the disease that is very different from your traditional OBG's. An acupuncturist looks at the many manifestations of endometriosis (pain during menstruation, pain before or after menstruation, low back pain, and the other symptoms, as well as what has worked in the past to alleviate your symptoms), and will make what is called a differential diagnosis. (This term also is used in traditional medicine but it means something entirely different.) This diagnosis may require a number of different treatments or needle placements.

One of the most significant ways in which acupuncture can have a positive effect on endometriosis is pain relief. If you are in severe pain and do not want to take as many analgesic drugs as you have been, you might do well to see an acupuncturist.

Chiropractic Spinal Manipulation

Chiropractic spinal manipulation has been pooh-poohed by traditional medical practitioners for decades, but it may be the best treatment for some types of back pain. Chiropractic holds that back problems (and other body dysfunction) stem from a misalignment of the vertebrae which can be corrected by physical adjustment. If this is indeed your problem, you might find relief in a chiropractor's office, but not for anything else. The spinal column has *no causative connection* with any other ailment. Chiropractic cannot help things such as allergies, digestive problems, cancer, high blood pressure, diabetes—or endometriosis.

However, if you think your backaches are not due as much to the endometrial lesions as to stress, a visit to a chiropractor might help. It can't hurt, and you will soon find out whether the spinal manipulations have helped.

One further word of warning about chiropractic: Do *not* seek this type of treatment if you have a herniated disk. Manipulating the vertebrae in the presence of this condition can do serious damage to the spinal nerves.

Massage

Massage is another way to create deep relaxation. In addition, it can improve joint range of motion, blood circulation, and generally enhance a sense of well-being. Be warned, though, that if you have blood clots, phlebitis, a skin disease, contusions, or infections, massage can exacerbate them.

In terms of endometriosis, a long, deep massage may be just what you need to relieve the stress of having the disease and going through the rigors of treatment. But tell the masseur or masseuse to stay away from your abdomen if you're in pain.

Naturopathy

Naturopathy can be helpful in that it emphasizes a healthy lifestyle (eating a nutritious diet, quitting smoking, reducing stress, and the like), but its belief that many illnesses can be cured by purging the body of impurities is bunk. A naturopath can do absolutely nothing for your endometriosis, and you are better off buying a book on nutrition than shelling out your hard-earned money (that will not be reimbursed by your health insurer) for naturopathy.

Herbal Medicine

Herbal medicine, the use of various plant leaves, stems, roots, and seeds to cure ills, is as old as human life on earth. Because herbal remedies contain such complex ingredients, there is no way to accurately test them for safety and efficacy (and for this reason, one should look at them askance), but some have been known to make people feel better—or think they feel better, which is much the same thing. Moreover, some well-tested and commonly accepted medications started out as herbal remedies, for example, digitalis for heart disease, rauwolfia for hypertension, and aspirin for aches and pains.

In Chinese medicine, certain herbs are thought to regulate and mimic the action of natural hormones, as well as bring the hormonal system into balance. If this is correct, there might be some benefit for endometriosis sufferers. Again, it probably can't hurt to try.

Some women with endometriosis find that herbal and other remedies can ease symptoms. For example:

- Vitamin E provides relief of the frequency and severity of the hot flashes that often occur as a result of natural menopause or oophorectomy. Although it is hard to get enough vitamin E from natural sources to create a therapeutic effect, foods that are good sources of the vitamin are wheat germ, wheat germ oil, safflower oil, whole grain breads and cereals, peanuts, walnuts, filberts, and almonds. A more efficient way to get a therapeutic dose of vitamin E is to take it in pill form at a dose of 800–1600 units a day.

- Ginseng is a potent source of plant estrogen, which seems to have the same effect as the animal or synthetic hormone. However, you never know how much estrogen you are getting with ginseng (and it is unopposed estrogen, that is, not tempered with progesterone) so you'll never know if you are taking an overdose.

• Garlic and other herbs, such as chamomile, catnip, hops, and passion flower, sometimes help with the symptoms of menopause. Taken in moderation (an occasional cup of tea), they probably can't hurt you, and they may even help.

If you do take herbal remedies, read the label carefully and try to find out if the manufacturer is reputable. You can call the FDA Division of Over-the-Counter Drugs, and there may be someone there who will talk to you about the manufacturer, but the remedies themselves do not fall within that agency's jurisdiction. Also, don't be surprised if the directions tell you to take six, eight, or even ten pills at a time. Herbs are far less purified than the chemicals we know as medications, and the pills often contain a proportionately larger amount of binder such as cellulose, starch, sugar, and other pharmacologically inactive ingredients.

Treatments That Can Cause Serious Harm

Chelation Therapy

Chelation therapy, whose practitioners claim that it is an acceptable alternative to cardiac bypass surgery and will cure a variety of other serious illnesses, is highly dangerous. The only legitimate use for chelation therapy, which is an intravenous infusion of chemicals designed to flush metal out of the body, is in lead poisoning. However, this should be done only in a hospital (usually in the emergency room) under the care of traditional physicians experienced in its use.

It's unlikely that you will find yourself in the office of someone who practices chelation therapy, but if you do and if the practitioner suggests that it can benefit your endometriosis, make tracks for the door in a hurry.

Dietary Supplements

Certain dietary supplements, if taken in sufficient quantity, can cause serious illness or kill. At best, they do nothing. For example, taking amino acids will not build muscle, increase intelligence, or treat insomnia. Large doses of vitamin A will not improve your vision; rather they can cause liver damage and birth defects. Megadoses of vitamin B₆ have been associated with nerve damage, and too much niacin causes nausea, vomiting, diarrhea, and liver damage. And the once-popular L-tryptophan, touted to relieve insomnia, killed 387 people, and hundreds of others suffered from crippling muscle pain.

The FDA does not guarantee the safety and efficacy of any of these dietary supplements; it is trying to crack down on their manufacture. It is against the law to sell any product for which a health claim is made unless it has been approved by the FDA, but manufacturers have devised a number of cunning ways to evade FDA inspectors and federal marshals.

Some women believe that dietary supplements in the form of vitamins and minerals can be of benefit in endometriosis, menopause, and other "female troubles." This is not true, and even if you suffer no physical harm, you will have wasted your money. If you eat a well-balanced diet and follow the U.S. Public Health Service guidelines described in chapter 5, you probably will get *all* the vitamins and minerals you need.

Instrumentation

Alternative health practitioners sometimes try to snow people with a variety of electric and mechanical devices which they claim have magical healing powers. Federal marshals seize these products when and where they can, but as always, there are more bad guys than good guys in the criminal arena, so there are still thousands of these machines out there in "doctors'" offices.

The only mechanical devices that will benefit endometriosis were described in chapter 4, and are used by licensed physicians, not alternative healers.

High Colonics

High colonic irrigation, a procedure in which as many as twenty gallons of water are pumped into the intestines through a tube inserted into the rectum, has been prescribed as a method to cleanse the body of its impurities. But the body's own organs—liver, kidneys, and intestines—are designed to do this job, so leave them alone and let them get on with it.

For women with endometriosis, a colonic irrigation could be particularly painful or damaging if there are endometriomata on the large intestine. If you are constipated, take a gentle laxative at bedtime or use a Fleet's enema.

Treatments That Are Useless But Harmless

Aromatherapy

Aromatherapy, an ancient Chinese form of herbal medicine that claims to cure various ills with aromatic plant oils, may smell pleasant and put one in a better mood, but it does not change physical health.

Bee Pollen

Bee pollen has been promoted for treatment of obesity, high blood pressure, arthritis, and more recently—and with lots of publicity—multiple sclerosis. There is no evidence to support any health claims for bee pollen.

Crystals

You may want to wear crystals around your neck on a chain or dangling from your earlobes because they look pretty, but they exert no aura and have no effect on the body.

Reflexology

Reflexology is massage that claims to treat illness and keep the life force in balance—whatever that means. Foot massage has been touted to govern energy channels—whatever they are. A nice massage is relaxing and a good stress reducer, but it has no other health benefits.

Homeopathy

Homeopathy is a technique that treats disease with tiny doses of natural substances that in larger amounts would cause the same symptoms as the disease. The theory is that these substances help the body heal itself by boosting natural defenses. There is no evidence one way or the other that homeopathy does any good, but the substances are given in such a small amount that they probably won't hurt.

There is no logical reason to believe that homeopathy would have any effect at all on endometriosis, because the disease is not caused by an external substance.

11

Social Issues

Paying for Endometriosis

Health Insurance

Endometriosis can be an expensive disease, so you must have health insurance. If you work, you will probably buy it as part of your employer's benefit package. If your employer does not provide it, if you are self-employed, if you are ineligible to be a dependent of your husband's policy, or if you are unmarried, buy a policy yourself. You have two choices about *how* you buy health insurance: you can go it alone and buy an individual policy, or you can join an organization and become eligible for its group health benefits.

There are several types of health insurance. Fee-for-service insurance, sometimes called traditional or conventional plan health insurance, is based on payment of a premium in exchange for which some portion of health care expenses is reimbursed. The size of the portion and the type of expenses reimbursed vary widely depending on the plan purchased and the amount of the deductible. In a fee-for-service plan, the health care provider first bills the insurance company and then bills the patient for whatever is not covered (called balance billing). This is the type of plan in which the choice of health care practitioner is completely yours.

Health maintenance organizations (HMOs) are managed care insurance plans that an individual or family joins as a dues paying member for a flat monthly or quarterly fee. The member receives almost all health care at no or little additional cost. Most HMOs charge a small per-visit fee in order to discourage unnecessary trips to the doctor. An HMO insists that you use one of its staff physicians as your primary care doctor who then refers you to a specialist if the primary (also known as the gatekeeper) thinks you require it. Your choice of health care practitioner is limited, and HMOs are extremely concerned about keeping health care costs down.

A preferred provider organization (PPO) is another type of controlled managed care plan whereby physicians and other health care providers arrange with an insurer to discount their fees. Providers are then paid by the insurer, with patients paying a small per-visit fee. If you are a member of a PPO, you receive full coverage if you choose a physician from the preferred list. If you choose an "outside" physician, you will pay most of the bill yourself. You also may be penalized by losing future benefits.

Medicare is a federal program, enacted by an amendment to the Social Security Act, that provides hospital and medical care coverage for people age sixty-five and older, as well as for some individuals who have been disabled for more than twenty-four months. Medicare is a government entitlement for which you have been paying taxes. It is *not* charity.

Medicaid is a joint federal-state program, also created by the Social Security Act, that provides health services for people who live at or below the federal poverty level and have no other way to pay for health care. Eligibility requirements and services provided vary from state to state. It too is funded by tax revenues.

Using COBRA When Changing Jobs

COBRA stands for Consolidated Omnibus Budget Reconciliation Act, but no one ever calls it that. COBRA is a federal law that protects you when you leave your job, whether you quit or were fired, so that for eighteen months, or until you find another job with health insurance benefits, you may participate with full coverage in the health insurance plan of the job you left. You will have to pay the premiums yourself, and the carrier (health insurance company) may charge you up to 2 percent more than it charges the employer, but this is always cheaper than buying an individual policy.

Once you leave your job, you have sixty days to sign up for COBRA benefits, but it is best to do it right away. Even if you are moving on to another job immediately, take the COBRA benefits because there may be a waiting period of one to six months before you are eligible for health insurance benefits on your new job. Even if you are eligible right away, what if you fall and break your leg over the weekend between the old job and the new one?

If you are disabled, your COBRA coverage can be extended to twenty-nine months, but you may not be able to make a case that endometriosis alone, which really has no disabling complications, constitutes a disability.

If after eighteen months, you have not found a job, you may be eligible for something called a conversion policy. This means that when your COBRA coverage runs out, the carrier will offer to cover you on the same policy—at a much larger premium, of course. About thirty-five states require insurers to offer conversion policies. When the offer is made, you have thirty days to respond.

Managed Care

Everyone has heard the term *managed care* by now, and, almost everyone hates it, but it is the most rapidly growing segment of the health care payment system in the United States.

HMOs are the purest form of managed care, although all health insurance plans now use some type of managed care system. More than 70 million Americans are enrolled in HMOs, and 95 percent of all employee health care benefits are under some type of managed care. In addition, Medicare and Medicaid are moving toward managed care payment systems.

Although managed care is a complex system of paying for health care, it can briefly be summarized as an arrangement whereby someone is interposed between patients and health care providers. This someone has the authority to place restrictions on how and from whom patients may receive services and what services are to be provided in any given situation.

Moreover, this person is not your health professional; it is usually an employee of an insurance company or health maintenance organization. In very broad strokes, here's how it works:

You go to your physician who makes a decision about the type of health care you require. But that decision is not final; unless it is an emergency, your health insurance company will have to approve what the physician wants to do.

In reality, things aren't as bad as this makes it sound. Physicians don't have to make a phone call for every little thing they do because insurance companies have devised lists of what they believe are appropriate procedures and treatments for various ailments. These are the things for which the insurance carrier will reimburse you, your physician, or other health care provider. For more out of the ordinary procedures or treatments, you will need to obtain approval from the carrier. It's a nuisance and that's what everyone—providers and their patients—hates.

However, managed care was instituted for a reason, and it has had some positive fallout for both physicians and patients, women in particular. Health care costs in the United States have been escalating beyond all reason, far outstripping all rates of inflation. In addition, there are almost 50 million Americans who have no health insurance at all (not even Medicare and Medicaid) and who have to pay for everything out of their own pockets—or go without care.

One of the reasons why health care costs so much is that so many physicians prescribe inappropriate and unnecessary procedures and treatments. They do this for two major reasons: plain old greed and a perceived need to practice "defensive medicine."

The first motivation needs no explanation, but you may not know what defensive medicine is. The incidence of medical malpractice lawsuits has escalated so dramatically in the past few decades that physicians are perpetually terrified of being sued, so they perform every diagnostic test and procedure they can think of in an effort to cover all bases, and to prove to the plaintiff's lawyers that they did everything reasonable and possible in the care of the patient suing. OBGs have been among the worst offenders in the practice of defensive medicine.

Medical malpractice suits, both reasonable and frivolous, have reached epidemic proportions, and health insurance companies had to foot the bill to pay for these defensive (and usually medically unnecessary) procedures. They have no way to control who sues a physician, but they do have control over what they will and will not reimburse. So they started clamping down and instituting much more stringent reimbursement policies.

Now, if physicians tell their patients to come to the office for this or that diagnostic procedure for endometriosis, and if they do a few office procedures or an outpatient laparoscopy, as well as prescribe medication ordinarily used to treat the disease, the insurance carrier will reimburse with no questions asked, because that is standard care for diagnosing and treating endometriosis. But if a physician wants patients to have a stress test in the absence of cardiac symptoms or a brain scan when they have not complained of anything wrong with their head, the carrier will say "No way!" Those tests would be unnecessary and inappropriate.

Insurers manage health care costs in four general ways:

- Physicians and other providers are given financial incentives to use fewer services and to discourage patients from overusing services. For women with endometriosis, this might mean that your primary care physician might discourage you from seeing an OBG once the diagnosis was made and treatment instituted.

- Managed care organizations designate certain providers who will give necessary care at the least cost; the practice patterns of these providers are closely monitored by the organization, especially the number of referrals to specialists.

- Insurance policies control and limit the services for which a managed care organization will pay. This means that if you want to go to a pain control clinic or nutritionist, for example, you may not be reimbursed.

- Various mechanisms discourage enrollment of high-risk patients with preexisting conditions such as endometriosis. Care of women with endometriosis costs more than caring for women without the disease; therefore, insurers will try their hardest to keep you off their rolls and may use a variety of unethical and illegal tactics to do so.

Some other ways in which managed care companies oversee health care costs include:

- except in emergencies, requiring approval before a patient is admitted to a hospital

- conducting ongoing reviews of patients' treatment

- day-to-day management of cases that require long-term and/or expensive care

- review of discharged hospital patients' medical records to determine the quality and necessity of all procedures and other elements of care

American consumers of health care, especially women, have benefited by not being subjected to unnecessary tests and treatments. All procedures carry risk and often have serious side effects. The less we are exposed to unnecessary risk, the better off we are, and the better off we are for not having to pay for something we didn't need in the first place.

Physicians hate managed care. First, they can no longer get away with performing as many expensive procedures as they used to, and medical procedures are their most profitable source of income. Second, they hate having to ask permission to do what they have been trained to do. Most physicians with busy practices have had to hire people who do nothing all day long but deal with insurance companies. This is expensive.

Managed care is generally unpleasant, but it will be good for American society in the long run. Anything that brings down the cost of providing health care, but doesn't lower the quality of that care, is desirable. The problem is determining whether managed care organizations, which include every health insurance carrier in the country, have taken so many cost-cutting steps that they have indeed jeopardized quality of care in some instances.

In Extreme Poverty

Endometriosis can be an expensive disease, even without surgery or a variety of complications, and if you are experiencing a severe case of the shorts, you might be tempted to suffer in silence and not get medical care. Don't. There are too many avenues of help for you to have to resort to jeopardizing your health.

There are a number of government, nonprofit, and voluntary clinics and other organizations, some of which are supported by pharmaceutical companies and other private industries, that provide free or low-cost care for women's health problems. It takes some time and effort to find them, but a few hours on the telephone should net you good results. Turn to the Resources section in the back of this book for suggestions of where to begin.

It's difficult, but have a frank discussion about money with your physician. You may be able to obtain free samples of whatever medication you are taking. If your doctor doesn't volunteer or doesn't have any samples, contact the pharmaceutical company yourself and explain your situation. They all have toll-free phone numbers for their customer relations department, and chances are, your request will be dealt with positively.

Next, call your state or county welfare office and find out if you are eligible for Medicaid and/or food stamps. In most states, if you earn more than $200 or $300 a month, you don't qualify, but it's worth a phone call. If you receive Aid to Families with Dependent Children (AFDC), Old Age Assistance (OAA), Aid to the Blind, Aid to the Permanently and Totally Disabled, or Supplemental Security Income (SSI), you will probably qualify for Medicaid.

The Veterans Administration, which operates the largest health care system in the United States, serves veterans in two major categories: those who have service-related health problems and those who are indigent. You may qualify in the latter category. Call or visit your local VA office to find out.

Employment Discrimination

Legally, your employer cannot discriminate against you if have endometriosis. Sooner or later, however, you may find yourself in a bind if you have missed too much work as a result of the disease. For instance, if you seriously exceed your employer's allotment of sick days, usually no more than ten to fourteen days a year, the issue becomes whether you can claim short-term disability because of endometriosis. You'll have to figure out how you will handle the consequences if your boss does not allow you to claim a disability, or what you'll do if you are fired because you are considered an unreliable employee.

Federal laws are your primary lines of defense against job discrimination. The Americans with Disabilities Act of 1990 protects people in private employment (businesses with more than fifteen employees), and the Federal Rehabilitation Act of 1973 offers the same protection for federal employees and people who work for companies that receive federal funding. In addition, there is a variety of state, county, and local laws that protect you against discrimination. The only problem is that it is unclear whether endometriosis falls into the category of protected diseases and conditions.

You probably don't think of yourself as disabled, and you shouldn't, but a good lawyer might be able to interpret these laws as including women with endometriosis in the definition of disabled, which includes "anyone who has a physical or mental impairment that substantially limits one or more major life activities, has a history of such impairment, or is regarded as having such an impairment." There are a number of ways in which these laws protect you at work:

- An employer cannot exclude you from its group health insurance plan. If you work at a place where there are fewer than fifteen employees, you can be required to undergo a health screening examination, which may or may not include a pelvic examination.

- An employer cannot ask you for health or medical information until you are offered a job, and only if it asks all employees the same questions.

- Once you have started working, your employer may not ask medical questions unless it is related to your job performance.

- An employer is required to provide reasonable physical accommodations for people with disabilities such as wheelchair ramps and wide doorways. For a woman with endometriosis, these accommodations *might* include additional sick leave without jeopardizing her job. Then again, they might not.

- If you lie when asked a legally permissible question about your health, you lose the protection of the law.

These laws and the benefits they provide mean a great deal to people with disabilities. They are an enormous step forward in providing equity to people who had been discriminated against for decades. However, for people with conditions that may or may not be considered a disability (such as endometriosis), things are not at all simple. First, the definitions of *disability* and *impairment* are at issue. Second, if you work in a place where there are fewer than fifteen employees, you're just plain out of luck—unless you have a really great boss. Third, if you decide to fight whatever discrimination you have been subjected to, you won't get far without a lawyer, and you don't need to be reminded how expensive they are.

In general, most attorneys will tell you that there are three steps in fighting discrimination: education, for which you don't need a lawyer; negotiation, for which you may or may not need a lawyer, depending on how much work you want to do yourself and how confident you feel about your ability to make your own case; and litigation, for which you definitely need a lawyer.

It is not within the scope of this book to go into detail about how to fight discrimination, or whether you ought to consider endometriosis a "real" disability; you need to consult an attorney for that, or talk it over with the federal Equal Employment Opportunities Commission. The problem with that agency is that it is filled with federal government bureaucrats who have a limited notion of what they do not know and cannot see. Endometriosis falls into this category; it doesn't show on the outside, and hardly anyone knows what it is. If you were wheelchair bound or walking around with a guide dog, you'd have no problem proving your case. But endometriosis is a difficult disease to describe and understand, and most women don't like the idea of sitting in the office of a stranger and describing their most intimate gynecologic problems. So the EEOC is probably not your best bet.

Sexual Activity

At some time or another, endometriosis will most likely have a negative effect on your sex life. If sex hurts, you're not going to want to do it. This will create a number of problems that you need to deal with, but there are ways to solve them.

Pain during intercourse arises from two major sources. The first is irritation of vaginal endometriomata, and the second is psychological. The remedy for the first is to treat the disease because if you have endometrial lesions in or near your vagina, intercourse will hurt.

The remedy for the second is a little harder to deal with. If you have had endometriosis for a long time, you're probably nervous and tense when contemplating sex, and as a result you feel turned off and skittish about having your husband or lover initiate lovemaking. Even if you *want* to have sex, your body may say "no" by drying up your vaginal mucosa and creating a bad atmosphere for sex. You can use K-Y jelly or Astro Glide for lubrication, but a much better remedy is to treat the endometriosis, wherever it is in your pelvic region, so that the very thought of sex doesn't make you think of pain.

Sexual intercourse does not hurt all the time, of course, so when you feel fine, take advantage of it. No couple, except those in the very first throes of passionate love, makes love all the time. Deep penetration during intercourse is the most common cause of sexual pain. To counteract it, learn which positions are most comfortable and use them (try lying side to side, or you assume the top position). If you need to, buy a manual on sex techniques and use it as a text. If you haven't done it so far, expand your sexual horizons to include activities other than intercourse.

Talk frankly with your husband or lover about what you like and don't like, what hurts and what doesn't, and how both of you feel about the effect of endometriosis on your sex life. Try to increase the level of emotional intimacy you share with one another. If he is not willing to talk about these things, if he makes fun of you, or if he insists on having sex when you have said you don't want to because you don't feel well, your marriage or relationship is in trouble in ways other than what transpires in the bedroom. You may want to rethink spending the rest of your life with such a man.

There are many stories of men who have used their wives' endometriosis as an excuse to have an affair with another woman: "Well, honey, if you're not going to give me what I need, I'll have to go out and find it somewhere else." This is unacceptable and extremely hurtful on a number of obvious levels, and if it has happened to you, you need to do something about it; try marriage counseling, family therapy, or simply putting your foot down and telling him to stop acting like a jerk.

Teach your husband or lover about endometriosis and why certain sexual activities hurt more than others. It's safe to say that the majority of men have no idea what endometriosis is (they've probably never heard the word), but many are amenable to learning. Take him with you when you next visit your OBG if you think that is appropriate.

If all else fails, get help from a sex therapist. Be careful, though, in whom you choose. Many sex therapists are phonies or voyeurs who get their jollies from talking about sex and listening to others describe their sexual activities. Many reputable sex therapists are licensed and certified psychotherapists so be sure you ask to see their credentials as you shop for a sex therapist. You also can call the American Association of Sex Educators, Counselors and Therapists in Chicago for a referral.

12

Medical Research

One of the many problems and frustrations of endometriosis is that so little definitive medical research has been conducted. Most of what is now known about the disease has been learned from observation, trial-and-error research, or anecdotal research rather than a more rigorous type of study.

Federally Funded Research

It is not likely that this situation will improve in the near future. For instance the National Institutes of Health (NIH), National Institute on Child Health and Human Development, the one that conducts research on women's health issues, has only four currently funded projects on endometriosis.

The first, at the Fred Hutchinson Cancer Research Center in Seattle (Holt, 1997), is looking at reproductive and contraceptive risk factors in endometriosis. Scientists at the Hutchinson Center acknowledge that few modifiable risk factors exist for endometriosis. Most of the studies that have attempted to identify such factors have been limited by the use of cases in which women were clearly infertile. Because these women may not be typical of all women with endometriosis, researchers at Fred Hutchinson are doing a study of endometriosis among all the women of reproductive age (about 750 women of all races) enrolled in a health maintenance organization. Their hypothesis is that spontaneous abortion (miscarriage) and induced abortion may increase the risk of endometriosis because of possible hormonal and immunologic influences.

The second study is taking place at the University of Missouri at Columbia (Sharpe, 1997). There, researchers are looking at two progesterone-induced uterine proteins. The hypothesis is that endometrial lesions found outside the uterus, although physiologically similar, are biochemically different from normal endometrium located inside the uterus—where it is supposed to be. The altered biochemical characteristics of the endometriomata may be involved with abnormalities of the immune system, ovulation, fertilization, and implantation, all of which have been implicated in infertility associated with endometriosis.

Using rats as a model for humans, scientists have isolated and identified two proteins that have been associated with endometriosis. The goal of the research is to purify and characterize both the rat and human forms of the proteins and to examine their structure and physiologic function in reproduction in general and endometriosis in particular.

In the third study, scientists at Reprogen, Inc., a company in Irvine, California (Snyder, 1997), are looking at autoantibodies to the endometrium. Autoimmunity is a malfunction of the body's immune system in which certain of the body's own substances (protein antigens) are mistakenly identified as "foreign invaders" and are attacked by the immune system. Because endometriosis may be linked to an abnormal autoimmune function, researchers at Reprogen want to isolate and characterize endometrial autoangitens that may react with autoantibodies to cause an autoimmune disease. If specific autoantigens can be identified and implicated in endometriosis, clinical assessment will be easier and more accurate, and physicians will gain a better understanding of infertility in endometriosis.

Fourth, scientists at the University of North Carolina at Chapel Hill (Lessey, 1997) are looking at endometrial integrins and uterine receptivity to a fertilized ovum. Integrins are cell adhesion molecules present in virtually all cells in the body that are active in many cell functions. The hypothesis is that integrins specific to menstrual cycle changes are implicated in embryo-endometrial interactions, that is, the way the endometrium responds to the presence of a fertilized ovum. If there is a dysfunction in this interaction, the ovum would have trouble implanting on the endometrium, making the woman infertile. Therefore, identifying a pattern of integrin expression may identify women at risk for infertility caused by defects in endometrial receptivity.

Possible Causes

NIH is not the only place where research on endometriosis is taking place. At the University of Oxford (UK) John Radcliffe Hospital, the Oxford Endometriosis Gene (OXEGENE) Study is underway. Scientists there believe that genetic susceptibility may play a role in the disease. Using new molecular biology techniques to identify genes may lead to better understanding of the causes of endometriosis. This type of research is called *linkage analysis* or *reverse genetics*.

One hypothesis is that endometriosis is multifactorial; that is, a number of genes interact with each other and with environmental factors such as exposure to dioxins or irradiation to increase the chance (not necessarily the inevitability) of a woman developing endometriosis.

The aim of the OXEGENE study is to identify susceptibility genes for endometriosis using linkage analysis (Kennedy, 1994). The technique involves collecting blood from sisters with surgically confirmed moderate to severe endometriosis, as well as blood from their parents, for DNA analysis. The first step in the link is to find tiny portions of chromosomes inherited from the parents of the affected sisters. The second step is to isolate individual genes from the chromosomes. So far, the Oxford group has contacted 435 families including more than 700 affected women. If you are interested in participating in this study, contact OXEGENE at its web site: www.medicine.ox.ac.uk/ndog/.

Environmental exposure to dioxin, found in many common herbicides and pesticides, may contribute to a rise in endometriosis rates. In studies conducted at the University of Wisconsin, Madison (Denison, 1994) in the primate lab, monkeys exposed to relatively low levels of dioxin over a four year period were more likely than nonexposed monkeys to develop endometriosis (79 percent of the exposed monkeys developed the disease). The severity of the disease was directly proportional to the dose of dioxin, and even monkeys who were exposed to the lowest dose of dioxin had a significantly increased incidence of endometriosis. Two of the monkeys died of the disease.

Moreover, the monkeys who had dioxin added to their diets had a hard time reproducing, and the offspring they produced had behavioral and other problems. Other studies have been done in mice and rats.

Dioxin is a toxic byproduct associated most frequently with medical and municipal incinerators, pesticides, and bleached pulp and paper products. It binds with hormone receptors, thus blocking their function. This in turn causes stymied or distorted sexual development in vulnerable embryos.

The specific dioxin chemicals that seem to have the highest causative association with endometriosis are 2,3,7,8-tetra chloro-dibenzo-p-dioxin (TCDD) and 2,3,4,7,8-pentachlorodi- benzofuran (4-PeCDF) (Cummings, Metcalf, et al., 1996). These are the chemicals that accumulate in the fatty tissue of animals and humans where they remain for years.

Although scientists don't fully understand the link between dioxin and endometriosis, and are therefore loath to recommend policy positions, one hypothesis is that chronic dioxin exposure may damage the immune system and thus increase the likelihood of endometriosis. It is, however, difficult to measure the potency of environmental chemicals and toxins and to assess their effect on animal and human biochemistry.

Potential New Treatments

Immunotherapy is a relatively new approach to treating endometriosis, although it was developed 4,000 years ago in China (Damewood, Kresch, and Metzger, 1997). The ancient Chinese didn't know, of course, about the immune system, but they did create a technique called oral tolerization.

In this technique, people are given a few drops under the tongue of a tiny amount of an antigen thought to contribute to the disease in question. If an allergic reaction develops, the treatment goal is to eliminate the reaction by building up the person's resistance to the antigen. In the case of endometriosis, several antigens may be culprits: estrogen, progesterone, luteinizing hormone, and a fungus called *Candida albicans*.

To determine which of these substances may produce an allergic reaction and to help determine dosage safe for treatment, a woman is given a skin test. If, within a few hours, the symptoms of endometriosis worsen, she is considered allergic to the organism or hormone and in need of treatment, which consists of oral tolerization, antifungal drugs, and nutritional corrections.

Women with mild to moderate endometriosis can be treated by immunotherapy alone (or in conjunction with other conservative medical therapy); those who have more severe disease also may require surgery. If immunotherapy alone is used, a woman can try to conceive because she maintains normal reproductive function.

There have been no scientifically designed clinical studies to determine the efficacy of immunotherapy, but in terms of anecdotal evidence, results have been positive. About 70 percent of women who have undergone immunotherapy have seen their symptoms diminish or even disappear. There are no known side effects, although recurrence of the disease is common after therapy is discontinued—as it is with more conventional therapy.

Resources

American Association of Acupuncture
and Oriental Medicine
    433 Front Street
    Catasauqua, Pa. 18032-2506
    610-433-2448

American Association of Biofeedback Clinicians
    2424 South Dempster Avenue
    Des Plaines, Ill. 60016
    312-827-0440

American Board of Medical Specialties
    47 Perimeter Center East, Suite 500
    Atlanta, Ga. 30346
    800-776-CERT

American Chronic Pain Association
    P.O. Box 850
    Rocklin, Calif. 95677
    916-632-0922

American College of Obstetricians and Gynecologists
    409 12th Street, S.W.
    Washington, D.C. 20024-2188
    202-638-5577

American Holistic Medical Association
  4101 Lake Boone Trail, Suite 201
  Raleigh, N.C. 27607
  919-787-5146

Endometriosis Association
  International Headquarters
  8585 North 76th Place
  Milwaukee, Wisc. 53223-2600
  800-992-3636

Holistic Health Hotline
  P.O. Box 25717
  Seattle, Wash. 98125
  206-481-4445

Infertility Awareness Association of Canada, Inc.
  396 Cooper Street, Suite 201
  Ottawa, Ontario K2P 2H7
  613-234-8585

International Foundation for Homeopathy
  2366 Eastlake Avenue, East, Suite 329
  Seattle, Wash. 98102
  206-324-8230

Medical Information Bureau (medical records)
  Consumer Information Office
  P.O. Box 105, Essex Station
  Boston, Mass. 02112
  617-426-3660

National Adoption Center
  1500 Walnut Street, Suite 701
  Philadelphia, Pa. 19102
  800-TO-ADOPT

National Chronic Pain Outreach Association
  822 Wycliffe Court
  Manassas, Va. 22110
  703-368-8884

National Commission for the Certification of
Acupuncturists
    1424 16th Street, N.W., Suite 105
    Washington, D.C. 20036
    202-232-1404

National Committee for Adoption
    3146 Connecticut Avenue, N.W., Suite 326
    Washington, D.C. 20008
    202-463-4825

National Health Information Center
    P.O. Box 1133
    Washington, D.C. 20013-1133
    800-336-4797

National Women's Health Network
    514 10th Street, N.W., Suite 400
    Washington, D.C. 20005
    202-347-1140

Public Citizen's Health Research Group
    2000 P Street, N.W., Suite 700
    Washington, D.C. 20036
    202-833-3000

Resolve (infertility issues)
    1310 Broadway
    Somerville, Mass. 02144-1731
    617-623-1156

Glossary

Acupuncture. A Chinese method of treatment whereby tiny needles are inserted into the skin at points that coincide with energy pathways known as meridians; puncture is said to open the flow of energy and keep it in balance throughout the body; often used to alleviate pain and for anesthesia.

Acute. Severity over a short period of time; usually refers to pain or disease.

Adenomyosis. A condition in which the endometrium grows into the muscular part of the uterus.

Adhesions. Bands of scar tissue that bind together normally separate tissue surfaces; usually a result of surgery.

Adrenal gland. A gland located atop each kidney that secretes hormones.

Amenorrhea. Absence of menstruation.

Analgesic. Drug or other substance that relieves pain.

Anaphylaxis. Severe, potentially fatal allergic reaction.

Androgen. Male sex hormone.

Anovulation. Failure to ovulate.

Antagonizing. Exerting an opposite effect.

Antibody. Part of the immune system; a cell that attacks a specific target known as an antigen.

Antigen. Any substance, most often a protein, that can cause formation of antibodies; signals the immune system to prepare to react.

Anus. The end of the alimentary canal; the point at which feces pass to the outside.

Artificial insemination. Insertion of sperm into the vagina by means other than sexual intercourse.

Aspiration (surgical). Puncture of a structure, usually a cyst, and suction of its contents; used for both biopsy and treatment.

Atrophy. Wasting away of tissue; decreasing in size.

Autoimmunity. A condition in which immune cells mistakenly sense the body's own tissue or cells as foreign and attack them; results in inflammation and various autoimmune diseases such as rheumatoid arthritis and lupus erythematosus.

Barium enema. Insertion through the rectum of a radiopaque dye into the lower bowel (colon) followed by X rays.

Benign. Not malignant.

Bilateral. Both sides.

Biopsy. Removal and microscopic examination of a piece of tissue in order to make a diagnosis.

Bladder. Sac that collects and stores urine.

Bowel. Intestine.

Broad ligaments. Folds of the peritoneum attached to the sides of the uterus.

Candidiasis. Infection by the yeast-like substance *Candida albicans*; commonly occurs in the vagina.

Carcinogenic. Capable of causing cancer.

Castration. Removal of the sex glands; oophorectomy in females.

Cauterize. Destruction of tissue by burning.

Cervix. The lowest part of the uterus; protrudes and opens into the vagina.

Chocolate cyst. Large benign tumor of endometrial tissue filled with old blood; seen most frequently on the ovaries.

Cholycystitis. Inflammation of the gallbladder.

Chronic. Of long duration and showing little change.

Coagulation. Clotting; process of changing a liquid to a solid, as in blood.

Colon. Large intestine; begins at the end of the small intestine and ends at the rectum.

Colonoscopy. Examination of the colon by means of a thin, flexible tube, with a fiberoptic light attached, inserted upward through the rectum.

Colposcopy. Visualization of the vagina and cervix through a magnifying device.

Colpotomy. Surgical procedure in which an incision is made in the vagina behind the cervix.

Congenital. Existing before birth; being born with.

Corpus luteum. A yellow glandular mass on the ovary formed from a mature ovarian follicle; produces progesterone during the second half of the menstrual cycle.

Cryosurgery. Destruction of tissue by freezing.

CT scan. Computerized tomography; computer-analyzed three-dimensional X ray examination of a layer of tissue.

Cul-de-sac. Space between the uterus and rectum that forms a pouch.

Cyst. Closed cavity or sac, usually containing liquid or semisolid material.

Cystitis. Inflammation of the bladder.

Cystoscopy. Examination of the bladder in which a tube, with a fiberoptic light attached, is inserted into the bladder through the urethra.

Dilatation and curettage (D&C). Stretching the cervix with instruments and then scraping the endometrium with surgical implements; used for diagnosis and to perform abortion.

Dissect. Cut apart or separate.

Dysfunction. Disturbance or abnormality in the normal function of tissue, organ, or system.

Dysmennorhea. Painful menstruation.

Dysparenunia. Painful sexual intercourse.

Dysplasia. Abnormal development of cells; possibly a precursor to cancer.

Dysuria. Painful urination.

Ectopic pregnancy. Implantation of a fertilized ovum in a location other than the uterus, commonly in a fallopian tube; a surgical emergency.

Electrocautery. Destruction of tissue by burning it with a wire heated by electric current.

Endocrine system. Network of glands (thyroid, pituitary, pancreas, ovaries, and testicles) and other structures that secrete hormones.

Endometrioma (plural: Endometriomata). Misplaced endometrial tissue.

Endometrium. Tissue that lines the uterus and builds up and sheds each month in response to hormonal stimuli.

Endorphins. Natural substances that diminish pain perception.

Estradiol. Major type of estrogen secreted during the menstrual years.

Estrogens. Female sex hormones.

Etiology. Cause.

Excise. To cut out.

Fiberoptic. Bundle of glass fibers that conducts light, used in surgical instruments to visualize parts of the body.

Fibroid. Noncancerous tumor of the body of the uterus; also called myoma (plural: myomyata) or leiomyoma.

Fibromyalgia. Painful condition of the connective tissue; sometimes seen in women with endometriosis.

Follicle. Clumps of cells in the ovary containing an immature egg.

Follicle stimulating hormone (FSH). Hormone produced in the pituitary gland, which with luteinizing hormone, stimulates the ovary to mature a follicle for ovulation.

Fornix. Area of the vagina that meets the cervix.

Fulguration. Destruction of tissue by burning by means of electrical sparks.

Gastrointestinal. Pertaining to the stomach and intestines.

Gonadotropins. Hormones produced by the pituitary gland that stimulate the sex glands.

Gonadotropin releasing hormone (GNRH). Substance produced in the hypothalamus that directs the pituitary to release follicle stimulating hormone and luteinizing hormone.

Hematuria. Blood in the urine.

Hormones. Chemical substances produced by the endocrine glands that regulate various body processes.

Histamine. Substance, sometimes a neurotransmitter, found in all body tissues that dilates small blood vessels and contracts smooth muscles; excess amounts are released during allergic reactions or shock.

Human chorionic gonadotropin (HCG). Hormone secreted by the placenta during pregnancy that maintains the corpus luteum and preserves the pregnancy.

Hyperparathyroidism. Abnormally increased activity of the parathyroid gland causing loss of calcium and phosphorus.

Hyperplasia. Abnormal multiplication of normal cells.

Hypertension. High blood pressure.

Hypotension. Low blood pressure.

Hypothalamus. A body attached to the pituitary gland that controls production and release of hormones in the pituitary.

Hysterectomy. Surgical removal of the uterus and cervix.

Hysterosalpingogram. Injection of dye into the uterus and fallopian tubes, followed by X ray.

Hysteroscopy. Insertion of a scope to visualize the interior of the uterus.

Incontinence. Inability to control urination; inadvertent loss of urine.

Infertility. Inability to conceive after one year of unprotected sexual intercourse.

Inguinal canal. Canal in the abdominal wall that contains the uterine round ligaments.

In situ. In the original position, e.g., cancer that has not metastasized.

Intestines. Tubular part of the digestive tract that extends from the stomach to the rectum through which digested food is passed; nutrients are absorbed from the small intestine, water is absorbed from the large intestine.

In vitro fertilization (IVF). A technique of artificial insemination used for women who have only part of an ovary; ova are retrieved from the body, fertilized by sperm in a petri dish, and reinserted into the uterus.

Labia. Folds of tissue at the entrance to the vagina.

Laparoscopy. Surgical procedure in which a small incision is made in or near the navel and a thin tube, with a fiberoptic light attached, is inserted into the abdominal cavity to visualize the contents; various instruments can be attached to the tube.

Laparotomy. Major abdominal surgery.

Laser. Highly concentrated beam of light used to repair or destroy tissue.

Lesion. In endometriosis, describes patches or colonies of misplaced endometrial tissue; also known as endometrioma.

Ligaments. Bands of elastic and muscle tissue that hold abdominal organs in place.

Luteal phase. The last fourteen days of the menstrual cycle during which the corpus luteum is formed and secretes progesterone.

Luteinization. Process by which the ovarian follicle becomes a corpus luteum.

Luteinizing hormone (LH). Secreted by the pituitary gland throughout the menstrual cycle and stimulates maturation of an ovarian follicle and release of an ovum.

Lymphatic system. A system of drainage and cleansing vessels running throughout the body, roughly parallel to the circulatory system; part of the body's defense against infection and disease; may be one means by which endometriosis spreads.

Lysis. Surgically cutting up, breaking or dividing.

Macrophage. White blood cell that serves as a cleansing agent in the blood; scavenger cell.

Malignant. Cancerous.

Menarche. Onset of menstruation.

Menopause. Cessation of menstruation.

Menorrhagia. Excessive prolonged menstrual flow.

Menorrhalgia. Difficulty during menstruation, including premenstrual distress, pelvic pain, and dysmenorrhea.

Menstruation. Cyclic shedding of the endometrium.

Metabolism. Chemical processes of a living organism that result in growth, energy production, and other body functions related to distribution of nutrients.

Metorrhagia. Bleeding between periods.

Myomectomy. Surgical removal of myomata.

Myometrium. Outer, muscular layer of the uterus.

Narcotic. Analgesic drug that has a potential for addiction.

Necrosis. Tissue death, usually in a localized site as a result of disease.

Neoplasia. New, abnormal cell growth.

Neurotransmitter. A naturally occurring biochemical that sends impulses along neural pathways.

Nocturia. Urinary frequency at night.

Nodule. Small, firm lump of tissue.

Oophorectomy. Surgical removal of one or both ovaries.

Ovarian wedge resection. Partial removal of an ovary.

Ovary. Female sex gland that produces ova and manufactures estrogen and progesterone.

Ovulation. Monthly ripening and rupture of an ovum from its follicle.

Ovum (plural: Ova). Egg.

Pain receptor. Nerve endings distributed in superficial layers of skin and on certain deeper tissues; also called nocioceptor.

Palpate. To feel with the hands.

Pap test. Used to detect abnormal cells, most frequently in the cervix.

Parathyroid gland. Composed of small bodies and located near the thyroid gland; concerned mainly with metabolism and phosphorus production.

Pelvic congestion. Abnormal accumulation of blood in the pelvis.

Pelvic inflammatory disease (PID). Infection in the pelvic area caused by a variety of bacteria.

Perineum. Space between the vaginal opening and the anus.

Peritoneum. Thin membrane covering the walls of the abdomen and pelvis; the organs contained within the abdomen.

Pituitary gland. Located at the base of the brain; secretes, regulates, and stores a number of hormones that affect the thyroid and reproductive and other organs.

Polycystic ovarian disease. Simultaneous formation of many cysts on both ovaries; also called Stein-Leventhal syndrome.

Polymenorrhea. Menstrual cycle shorter than three weeks.

Posterior. In back of; behind.

Premature menopause. Occurring earlier than normal.

Presacral neurectomy. Severing nerves at the back of the uterus to provide pain relief.

Proctoscopy. Insertion of a lighted scope or speculum to examine the rectum.

Progesterone. Hormone that prepares the uterus for reception and development of fertilized egg.

Prostaglandin. Substance found in semen, menstrual fluid, and body tissues; contracts the uterus and other smooth muscles; can lower blood pressure and affect the action of certain hormones.

Pseudomenopause. Chemical stimulation of hormones to mimic menopause; a treatment for endometriosis.

Rectovaginal septum. Partition that separates the rectum and vagina.

Rectum. The end portion of the large intestine where feces are stored.

Resect. To excise part of an organ or other structure.

Retroflexed. Bent backward.

Retrograde menstruation. Backward flow of menstrual fluid through the fallopian tubes and into the pelvic cavity.

Retroperitoneal. Behind the peritoneum.

Retroverted. Tilted backward.

Round ligament. Band of tissue that suspends the uterus.

Salpingectomy. Removal of a fallopian tube.

Sigmoid colon. Lower part of the large intestine located in the pelvis and extending to the rectum.

Sigmoidoscopy. Insertion of a tube called a sigmoidoscope, with a fiberoptic light attached, through the rectum to examine the sigmoid colon.

Speculum. Instrument used to open or widen a passageway, most often the vagina, to view the contents.

Spontaneous abortion. Miscarriage.

Stenosis. Narrowing.

Steroids. Group of molecules with a common structure that includes sex hormones, cholesterol, bile acids, and other biologically active compounds.

Surgical menopause. Menopause brought about by surgical removal of ovaries.

Systemic. Pertaining to the body as a whole.

Tenaculum. Instrument used to seize and hold a body part, often the cervix.

Testosterone. One of a group of male hormones.

Tuboplasty. Surgical reconstruction of a fallopian tube.

Ultrasound. Translation of sound waves into a video image.

Ureter. Tube that carries urine from the kidneys to the bladder.

Urethra. Tube that carries urine from the bladder to the outside.

Uterine suspension. Shortening and repositioning of the uterine ligaments to hold the uterus up and out of the cul-de-sac in an attempt to prevent formation of adhesions.

Uterosacral ligaments. Bands of fibrous tissue that support the uterus.

Uterus. Pear-shaped muscular organ that holds and maintains the fetus during pregnancy.

Vagina. Canal connecting the external genitalia and the uterus.

Vaginismus. Muscle spasm at the opening of the vagina that hinders penetration during sexual intercourse.

Vaporization. Destruction of tissue by instant boiling of the water inside the cells with a laser or electrosurgical knife.

Visceral. Referring to abdominal organs.

Bibliography

American College of Obstetricians and Gynecologists. 1993. *Endometriosis.* Technical Bulletin No. 184. Washington, D.C.: American College of Obstetrics and Gynecologists.

Ballweg, Mary Lou. 1995. *The Endometriosis Sourcebook.* New York: Contemporary Books.

Boston Women's Health Book Collective. 1992. *The New Our Bodies, Ourselves.* New York: Simon and Schuster.

Breitkopf, Lyle J., and Marion Gordon Bakoulis. 1994. *Coping with Endometriosis.* New York: Prentice Hall.

Brinton, L. A., G. Gridley, I. Persson, and A. B. Baron. 1997. Cancer risk after a hospital discharge of endometriosis. *American Journal of Obstetrics and Gynecology* 176:572

Buck, G. M., L. E. Sever, R. E. Batt, and P. Mendola. 1987. Life-style factors and female infertility. *Epidemiology* 8:435–41.

Campion, Edward W. 1993. Why unconventional medicine? *New England Journal of Medicine* 328:282–83.

Cummings, A. M., J. L. Metcalf, and L. Birnbaum. 1996. Promotion of endometriosis by 2,3,7,8-tetrachlorodibenzo-p-dioxin in rats and mice: time-dose dependence and species comparison. *Toxicology and Applied Pharmacology.* 138:131–9.

Damewood, Marian, Arnold J. Kresch, and Deborah Metzger. 1997. Current approaches to endometriosis. *Patient Care.* January, 34–44.

Dawood, M. Yusoff, Charles W. Obasiolu, Josefina Ramos, and Firyal S. Khan-Dawood. 1997. Clinical, endocrine and metabolic effects of two doses of gestrinone in treatment of pelvic endometriosis. *American Journal of Obstetrics and Gynecology.* 176:387–97.

Denison, Niki. 1994. From a candle to a flame. *On Wisconsin.* November/December, 24–52.

Dennerstein, Lorraine, Carl Wood, and Ann Westmore. 1995. *Hysterectomy: New Options and Advances.* New York: Oxford University Press.

Edmonds, D. K. 1996. Add-back therapy in the treatment of endometriosis: the european experience. *British Journal of Obstetrics and Gynaecology* 103 Suppl 14:10–3.

Eisenberg, David M. 1993. Unconventional medicine in the United States. *New England Journal of Medicine.* 328:246–52.

Fogel, Catherine Ingram, and Nancy Fugate Woods. 1981. *Health Care of Women.* St. Louis. The C. V. Mosby Co.

Goldfarb, Herbert A. 1990. *The No-Hysterectomy Option.* Baltimore: John Wiley and Sons.

Holt, Virginia L. 1997. *Reproductive/Contraceptive Risk Factors and Endometriosis.* Seattle: Fred Hutchinson Cancer Research Center.

Johnson, K. L., A. M. Cummings, and L. S. Birnbaum. 1997. Promotion of endometriosis in mice by polychlorinated dibenzo-p-dioxins, dibenzofurans, and biphenyls. *Environmental Health Perspectives* 105:750–55.

Kennedy, Stephen. 1994. The Oxford endometriosis gene (OXEGENE) study. *St. Charles Endometriosis Treatment Program Newsletter.* Winter, 1–3.

Lessey, Bruce A. 1997. Endometrial integrins and uterine receptivity. Chapel Hill: University of North Carolina at Chapel Hill.

Matalliotakis, I., M. Neonaki, A. Zolindaki, and E. Hassan, et al. 1997. Changes in immunologic variables (TNF-a, sCD8 and sCD4) during danazol treatment in patients with endometriosis. *International Journal of Fertility and Women's Medicine.* 42:211–4.

Orwoll, Eric S. 1994. Nafarelin therapy in endometriosis: Long-term effects on bone mineral density. *American Journal of Obstetrics and Gynecology.* 171:463–67.

Reprogen, Inc., Irvine, Calif. 1997. Abstract of research plan submitted to national institute of child health and human development. (unpublished).

Rier, S. E. and Martin, D. C. 1995. Immunosuppressiveness in endometriosis: implications of estrogenic toxicants. *Environmental Health Perspectives* 103 (suppl 7):151–156.

Sachs, Judith. 1991. *What Women Can Do About Endometriosis*. New York: Dell Publishing.

Schenken, Robert S. 1989. *Endometriosis: Contemporary Concepts in Clinical Management*. Philadelphia: Lippincott.

Sharpe, Kathy L. 1997. *Endometriosis-Associated Secretory Proteins*. Columbia, Mo.: University of Missouri at Columbia.

Sheppard, Bruce D., and Carroll A. Sheppard. 1982. *The Complete Guide to Women's Health*. Tampa: Mariner Publishing.

Smith, S. K. 1997. Angiogenesis. *Seminars on Reproductive Endocrinology* 15:221–7.

Snyder, Patrick A. 1995. *Characteristics of Autoantibody Reactive Endometrial Antigens*. Irvine, Calif: Reprogen, Inc.

Weinstein, Kate. 1987. *Living with Endometriosis*. New York: Addison-Wesley.

More New Harbinger Titles

HIGH ON STRESS
A Woman's Guide to Optimizing the Stress in Her Life
Helps you rethink the role of stress in your life, rework your physical and mental responses to it, and find ways to boost the positive impact that it can have on your well-being.
  Item HOS $13.95

PERIMENOPAUSE
Changes in Women's Health After 35
Perimenopause begins with subtle physiological changes in the mid-thirties and forties, and it can encompass a bewildering array of symptoms. This self-care guide helps you cope and assure your health and vitality in the years ahead.
  Item PERI $13.95

A WOMAN'S GUIDE TO OVERCOMING SEXUAL FEAR AND PAIN
Provides a series of exercises designed to help you map the terra incognita of your own body and begin to overcome fear or pain that blocks or inhibits your sexuality.
  Item WGOS $14.95

THE TAKING CHARGE OF MENOPAUSE WORKBOOK
Helps you ease the transition through this major life change by becoming an active member of your health care team.
  Item PAUS $17.95

PMS
Women Tell Women How to Control Premenstrual Syndrome
Draws on the experiences of more than 1,000 women to show how to break the vicious PMS cycle of anger, guilt, denial, and depression.
  Item PRE $13.95

THE FIBROMYALGIA ADVOCATE
Shows you how to assemble a functional health care team, deal with the legal aspects of the health care system, and fight for your right to receive effective care for fibromyalgia and the related condition of myofascial pain syndrome.
  Item FMA $18.95

Call **toll-free 1-800-748-6273** to order. Have your Visa or Mastercard number ready. Or send a check for the titles you want to New Harbinger Publications, 5674 Shattuck Avenue, Oakland, CA 94609. Include $3.80 for the first book and 75¢ for each additional book to cover shipping and handling. (California residents please include appropriate sales tax.) Allow four to six weeks for delivery.

Prices subject to change without notice.

Some Other New Harbinger Self-Help Titles

High on Stress: A Woman's Guide to Optimizing the Stress in Her Life, $13.95
Infidelity: A Survival Guide, $12.95
Stop Walking on Eggshells, $13.95
Consumer's Guide to Psychiatric Drugs, $13.95
The Fibromyalgia Advocate: Getting the Support You Need to Cope with Fibromyalgia and Myofascial Pain, $18.95
Healing Fear: New Approaches to Overcoming Anxiety, $16.95
Working Anger: Preventing and Resolving Conflict on the Job, $12.95
Sex Smart: How Your Childhood Shaped Your Sexual Life and What to Do About It, $14.95
You Can Free Yourself From Alcohol & Drugs, $13.95
Amongst Ourselves: A Self-Help Guide to Living with Dissociative Identity Disorder, $14.95
Healthy Living with Diabetes, $13.95
Dr. Carl Robinson's Basic Baby Care, $10.95
Better Boundries: Owning and Treasuring Your Life, $13.95
Goodbye Good Girl, $12.95
Being, Belonging, Doing, $10.95
Thoughts & Feelings, Second Edition, $18.95
Depression: How It Happens, How It's Healed, $14.95
Trust After Trauma, $13.95
The Chemotherapy & Radiation Survival Guide, Second Edition, $14.95
Heart Therapy, $13.95
Surviving Childhood Cancer, $12.95
The Headache & Neck Pain Workbook, $14.95
Perimenopause, $13.95
The Self-Forgiveness Handbook, $12.95
A Woman's Guide to Overcoming Sexual Fear and Pain, $14.95
Mind Over Malignancy, $12.95
Treating Panic Disorder and Agoraphobia, $44.95
Scarred Soul, $13.95
The Angry Heart, $14.95
Don't Take It Personally, $12.95
Becoming a Wise Parent For Your Grown Child, $12.95
Clear Your Past, Change Your Future, $13.95
Preparing for Surgery, $17.95
The Power of Two, $12.95
It's Not OK Anymore, $13.95
The Daily Relaxer, $12.95
The Body Image Workbook, $17.95
Living with ADD, $17.95
Taking the Anxiety Out of Taking Tests, $12.95
Five Weeks to Healing Stress: The Wellness Option, $17.95
Why Children Misbehave and What to Do About It, $14.95
When Anger Hurts Your Kids, $12.95
The Addiction Workbook, $17.95
The Chronic Pain Control Workbook, Second Edition, $17.95
Fibromyalgia & Chronic Myofascial Pain Syndrome, $19.95
Flying Without Fear, $13.95
Kid Cooperation: How to Stop Yelling, Nagging & Pleading and Get Kids to Cooperate, $13.95
The Stop Smoking Workbook: Your Guide to Healthy Quitting, $17.95
Conquering Carpal Tunnel Syndrome and Other Repetitive Strain Injuries, $17.95
An End to Panic: Breakthrough Techniques for Overcoming Panic Disorder, Second Edition, $18.95
Letting Go of Anger: The 10 Most Common Anger Styles and What to Do About Them, $12.95
Messages: The Communication Skills Workbook, Second Edition, $13.95
Coping With Chronic Fatigue Syndrome: Nine Things You Can Do, $13.95
The Anxiety & Phobia Workbook, Second Edition, $18.95
The Relaxation & Stress Reduction Workbook, Fourth Edition, $17.95
Living Without Depression & Manic Depression: A Workbook for Maintaining Mood Stability, $17.95
Coping With Schizophrenia: A Guide For Families, $15.95
Visualization for Change, Second Edition, $15.95
Postpartum Survival Guide, $13.95
Angry All the Time: An Emergency Guide to Anger Control, $12.95
Couple Skills: Making Your Relationship Work, $13.95
Self-Esteem, Second Edition, $13.95
I Can't Get Over It, A Handbook for Trauma Survivors, Second Edition, $15.95
Dying of Embarrassment: Help for Social Anxiety and Social Phobia, $13.95
The Depression Workbook: Living With Depression and Manic Depression, $17.95
Men & Grief: A Guide for Men Surviving the Death of a Loved One, $14.95
When Once Is Not Enough: Help for Obsessive Compulsives, $13.95
Beyond Grief: A Guide for Recovering from the Death of a Loved One, $13.95
Hypnosis for Change: A Manual of Proven Techniques, Third Edition, $15.95
When Anger Hurts, $13.95

Call **toll free, 1-800-748-6273,** to order. Have your Visa or Mastercard number ready. Or send a check for the titles you want to New Harbinger Publications, Inc., 5674 Shattuck Ave., Oakland, CA 94609. Include $3.80 for the first book and 75¢ for each additional book, to cover shipping and handling. (California residents please include appropriate sales tax.) Allow two to five weeks for delivery.

Prices subject to change without notice.